CHRONIC PAIN
Out-of-the-box Treatments that Cure

Lakshmi Champak Vas

Director, Ashirvad Institute for Pain Management and Research
Honorary Consultant Pain Medicine Seth GS Medical College and
King Edward Memorial Hospital Parel Mumbai
National Burns Centre Airoli Mumbai, India

CRC Press
Taylor & Francis Group
Boca Raton London New York

CRC Press is an imprint of the
Taylor & Francis Group, an **informa** business

A SCIENCE PUBLISHERS BOOK

First edition published 2024
by CRC Press
2385 NW Executive Center Drive, Suite 320, Boca Raton FL 33431

and by CRC Press
4 Park Square, Milton Park, Abingdon, Oxon, OX14 4RN

CRC Press is an imprint of Taylor & Francis Group, LLC

Library of Congress Cataloging-in-Publication Data (applied for)

ISBN: 978-1-032-56048-9 (hbk)
ISBN: 978-1-032-56049-6 (pbk)
ISBN: 978-1-003-43355-2 (ebk)

DOI: 10.1201/9781003433552

Typeset in Times New Roman
by Radiant Productions

Dedication

To my patients, my teachers

The universal spirit saw to it that I learnt from the best; it guided me to a maverick understanding of pain, which led to the evolution of highly effective treatments.

Foreword

Dr. Lakshmi Vas is a well-known name in the speciality of Pain Control and Pain Management in India.

She is known to me for over 25 years. Earlier as a reputed paediatric Anaesthetist and later as a Pain Care Specialist.

I am an ex-Professor of Orthopaedics, specialised in spine care and spine surgery. I am senior teacher and faculty, both nationally and internationally, for spine Surgery and Non-surgical spine care.

She was associated with me as a trainee in Skeletal Pain Management for over 3 years.

I know her as an academic minded Pain Care Specialist with continuous quest for knowledge. She is also a well-known, popular Teacher for Pain Care and draws students from India and other countries.

The author is a thinker medical practitioner. She diligently evaluates every patient and his/her problem, in detail and comes out with a tailor-made solution.

My experience of running the "Back School (the patient education program) over the last 35 years, is that, "to know everything about their acute or chronic Back and Neck pain is a compulsive need of most patients." Same is the case with pains of other areas and of other origin.

This book, Chronic Pain: Out-of-the-box Treatments that Cure written by Dr. Lakshmi Vas, exactly fulfils that need.

Amongst all such books, publications I have found this one to be the most comprehensive. She has used simple, everyday language and clearly but succinctly described every necessary aspect of pain and suffering.

The anecdotes, examples, metaphors she has used are from day-to-day life of everybody. Almost every reader will instantly know what she wants to convey and will understand the concepts and medical technical details.

This book is an excellent blend of the up-to-date scientific knowledge and the vast clinical experience of the author. She has holistic approach to the patient care and that is seen here.

Chronic pains are difficult to treat. They have contribution coming from mental and emotional disturbance. The book makes the reader understand this. The book also tells the reader why many pains become chronic, why they are difficult to treat and how a patient should participate and help the process of recovery.

The treatment protocols focus not only on treating the pain and its source, but also improve the secondarily affected body functions.

For whom Is this book? As on today, the basic curricula of medical students, therapy students and such, do not include sufficient deliberations about the pain phenomena, the pain production, the pain management etc. There are lots of grey areas in many peoples understanding the pain as a clinical entity, even though they are compelled to treat pain patients. Though this book is primarily aimed at common lay person, it goes beyond and contains sufficient detailed information for pain-care givers.

The book has high production value. The paper selection, the fonts, the editorial arrangement etc is professional. The textual content has been well supported and enhanced by the appropriate illustrations and diagrams.

Many books are for browsing or casual one-time reading. I think this book has an important place in every family's book-shelf. Because it has a practical value and people will refer to it now and then.

Prof. V T Ingalhalikar

- Ex Prof of Orthopaedics & Spine Surgery LTM Medical college, Mumbai.
- The founder and later President of Association of Spine Surgeons of India.
- Director of "Spine Clinic' , Jupiter Hospital Thane.
- Started the First exclusive Spine Clinic and the first Back School in India in 1984.

Preface

The evolution of this book spans 18 years, from early 2006, when the initial idea took root in my mind. During this time I began to witness what were previously considered 'incurable' conditions showing signs of improvement, which served as a catalyst for this project. I put pen to paper, however, only in 2013, with some thoughts and stories of patients' journeys. I was inspired to write a book on pain management for the public, but somehow there was always something else that came up. Over the past three decades, my professional life has been characterized by many dramatic, at times jerky and turbulent, at other times, uncertain twists and turns, but everything honed into the highest point of my life when I established Ashirvad Institute for Pain Management and Research in 2005. My centre is named 'Ashirvad' because it not only bestows the blessing of pain relief to patients but also is a singular blessing to me and my team, to enable it.

Till the turn of the century in 2000, as a leading paediatric anaesthesiologist in a major charitable children's hospital, I was content with the thought that I was serving society well. But only after I started chronic-pain management did I realize what a privilege it was to be of service to people suffering from chronic pain. By some lucky quirk of destiny, I was conferred the gift of a different perspective on pain. My success has been solely due to this different perspective, which led to my developing many new concepts and innovations, and this convinced me that pain management has to be rewritten from this new perspective. I had an obligation to patients, the world over, to share with them all that I have learnt from my patients. My objective is to assert that there is no need to suffer from chronic pain. No pain is hopeless. There is always some way to relieve pain—some completely, some partially, but it is always possible to reduce pain to a bearable level.

Then one fine day, I thought, why not let the patients' experiences speak for themselves? That would be authentic and unbiased. I can only add what treatment was given. Thus, this book details my learning curve, on the journey to becoming a pain specialist, and the birth of the blessing, 'Ashirvad' as we discovered and implemented the unique protocols, thanks entirely to the patients who vested their faith and confidence in me. I have described pain and the out-of-the box Ashirvad approach to pain management; how we treat our patients, the basis for our diagnoses, our perspective on the pain of a particular patient and the justification for the treatment given. Interspersed in many of the chapters, I have shared the in-depth learning I derived from my patients who became my teachers; how their confidence and cooperation motivated me to keep working to achieve the ultimate goal of pain relief. I have written about some unusual cases, and the challenges faced.

Through all the narratives, the patients have shared their pains; of how they went in vain from doctor to doctor looking for relief, till they came to Ashirvad. Some got there by sheer chance, some because a friend or relative recommended it, some through the website, and some via doctor referrals. In this text, we refer to our patients by random alphabets to protect their privacy.

Although I have written this book to acknowledge how my patients educated me in understanding pain and its management, it can certainly serve the purpose of educating patients about their access and right to managing pain. I have used initials and concealed references as far as possible, to ensure that their identity is not disclosed.

In the Preamble, I have described the details of my journey from paediatric anaesthesia to pain management and how it all started.

Lakshmi Champak Vas

Director, Ashirvad Institute of Pain Management and
Research (AIPMR)

Acknowledgements

My journey became possible because of the innumerable people who stood by me all the way. My family ungrudgingly gave up their time with me so that I could pursue my vocation. My parents instilled a reverence for humanity and work. My father considered work as a calling, and my mother had the simple policy, "Why at all would anybody come to you unless they have a need? And what better privilege than fulfilling that need?"

My friend, philosopher, and guide, Vasu, my husband, has always unconditionally supported me and made it his business to see that I became a pain specialist. My children have been my pride and joy and they made it their job description to regularly cut me down to size to ensure that I remained grounded in reality. My grandchildren put me in daily touch with the Almighty just by being their joyful selves.

My teachers allowed me to stand on their shoulders so that I could see beyond. My friends have always been there for me unconditionally. My staff has created an environment of empathy and care to all patients. My students never fail to share my wonderment at the success of the "out-of- the-box" Ashirvad concepts.

Dr Mary Abraham, my dear friend from Bangalore medical college, created the amazing illustrations for this book to prove the adage, "A picture is worth a thousand words." My student, Dr Khyati Patel, has added some more figures. Finally, Ms Indu Ramchandani, has painstakingly edited this book to whip it into shape.

Lakshmi Champak Vas

Contents

Glossary of Abbreviated Medical Terms

AIIMS	All-India Institute of Medical Sciences
AIIPMR	All-India Institute of Physical Medicine and Rehabilitation
AIPMR	Ashirvad Institute of Pain Management and Research
CBPB	Continuous brachial plexus block
CBT	Cognitive behavioural therapy
CDC	Clinical diagnostic criteria
CNB	Continuous nerve block
CNS	Central nervous system
COPD	Chronic obstructive lung disease
CRF	Continuous radiofrequency
CRPS	Complex regional pain syndrome
CSF	Cerebrospinal fluid
DASH	Disability of the arm, shoulder, and hand
DMARD	Disease modifying antirheumatic drug
DMSO	Dimethyl sulfoxide
DN	Dry needling
DRG Stim	Dorsal root ganglion stimulation
EMG	Electromyograph
FFF	Fright-fight-flight (or freeze) reflex
FM	Fibromyalgia
fMRI	functional magnetic resonance imaging
GAG	Glucosanaminoglycan
GP	General physician
IASP	International Association for the Study of Pain
IBS	Irritable bowel syndrome

ICS (also PBS)	Interstitial cystitis syndrome or painful bladder syndrome
IDDS	Intradural drug delivery systems
IFT	Interferential current treatment
IMS	Intramuscular stimulation
IPJ	Interphalangeal joints
ITP	Intrathecal pump
LCS	Lumbar canal stenosis
LTR	Local twitch reflex
MC	Modic changes
MCPJ	Metacarpophalangeal joints
MPS	Myofascial pain syndrome
MRI	Magnetic resonance imaging
MTrP	Myofascial Trigger Point
MUS	Medically unexplained symptom
NCV	Nerve conduction velocity
NICU	Neonatal intensive care units
NMJ	Neuromuscular junction
NRS	Numerical Rating Scale
NSAID	Non-steroidal anti-inflammatory drug
PAKH	Prince Alykhan Hospital
PHN	Postherpetic neuralgia
PNS	Peripheral nervous system
PRF	Pulsed radiofrequency
PTTN	Painful traumatic trigeminal neuropathy and neuralgia
RA	Rheumatoid arthritis
RF	Radiofrequency
RFA	Radiofrequency ablation
ROM	Range of movement
RSD	Reflex sympathetic dystrophy
SCS	Spinal cord stimulation/stimulators
SGB	Stellate ganglion block
SSF	Search faradic current
TENS	Transcutaneous electrical nerve stimulation
TFES	Transforaminal epidural steroid injection
USGDN	Ultrasound guided dry needling

Preamble
How It All Started

Human beings with all their achievements are so much the flotsam and jetsam in the meandering stream of life. Yet, when individual aims and aspirations coincide with the currents of universal direction, work takes on an impetus that is self-propelling and self-sustained as if moulded by an unseen hand. I realized this very early in my pain practice, which I entered after my sojourn as the head of paediatric anaesthesia at the Bai Jerbai Wadia hospital for children in Mumbai. The plunge from the heights of anaesthesia expertise to the unknown and uncharted depths of pain management was scarier than the bungee jump (Figure 1) that I did off the Kawarau bridge in Queenstown, New Zealand.

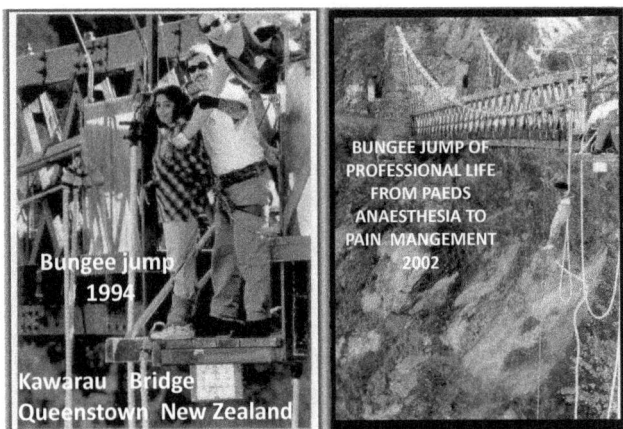

Figure 1

In early 2000, I was among the elite group of fewer than ten paediatric anaesthesiologists in India, specializing in anaesthetizing children, infants, and new-born babies. I was happily ensconced in this world, revelling in my role as an expert in this very esoteric and challenging specialization, teaching postgraduates the intricacies of this fascinating branch, and with their help, engaging in meaningful clinical research. This pioneering work in regional anaesthesia in children, was regularly published in international journals. Life was good! I was too busy with the academic high, travelling around the country lecturing and teaching, blissfully unaware of the *coup de grace* that fate had in store for me. The unprecedented changes that were brewing came to a head culminating in my resignation from Wadia Children's. I was rather bewildered and confused at the irony—here I was, an expert, who was providing pro-bono services, and Wadia, a hospital with resource crunches, needed honorary consultants. Yet situations had transpired to break this seemingly ideal combination!

After I left Wadia, I got busy in a lucrative private practice with my friend Ashok Johari, a paediatric orthopaedic surgeon. Thus, my work remained similar to Wadia Children's. A work schedule from 8.30 am till 8–9 pm, often going till 2 am the next morning, left no time to sustain the mind's devil's workshop! My work and the utter stability in my personal life with my family's support, propelled me beyond the Wadia phase. I also worked honorarily at the All-India Institute of Physical Medicine and Rehabilitation (AIIPMR), setting up modern anaesthesia practices. All this was most gratifying. In 1999, I attended the first Asian paediatric anaesthesia conference at the modern, superbly equipped and staffed KK hospital for women and children, in Singapore. After I presented my paper, Agnes Ng, the KK hospital anaesthesia chief, offered me a job! My family was supportive, the children very enthusiastic, so I accepted the offer only for six months. Working at KKH proved to be all that I had expected in India but had never been able to achieve. There were no struggles, no arguments with administrators for expensive safety equipment, all facilities and staff adequacy to ensure safe passage of my babies through anaesthesia, at all times! The safety standards were impeccable, the opportunities for clinical research absolutely unfettered with access to undreamt of resources. The icing on the cake was the lasting friendships. Yet, the irony of the situation hit me at every turn. Here I was, an outcast from the Indian system (recalling the traumatic exit from Wadia), welcomed in another country, which had bent many rules to get me, a doctor from a developing country with no 'foreign' qualifications, to work as a consultant. Yet, at the end of six months, when they offered a permanent position, I regretfully declined, convinced that my expert services were needed more in India than in affluent Singapore where they could get whomsoever they wanted.

I resumed work with Ashok in Mumbai but, there was a strange restlessness to teach and share my expertise. I looked for teaching positions, but the irony continued to haunt me. All doors of opportunities were getting shut in my face. In the meantime, my husband Vasu, who had been after me for decades to start a pain clinic, redoubled his urging. Whenever I said, "Look Vasu, although I can treat acute pain easily, I have no idea about chronic pain, there are no courses in India and nobody teaching them." His unsympathetic retort always was, "Who taught you paediatric anaesthesia?" Egging me on, "Take a sabbatical from work, read and teach yourself about pain, then go and observe what they do in pain clinics abroad. I will take care of finances."

Still, I vacillated and dithered at the thought of leaving the familiar, and more importantly, the beloved branch of paediatric anaesthesia. The final straw that broke the camel's back came in the form of a 'negative' input, a very innocuous but belittling comment about anaesthesia by a junior surgeon. That comment, possibly meant to be friendly ribbing of give and take, annoyed me inordinately and I decided, "This is it, no more anaesthesia work from tomorrow"! Immediately, I told Ashok that I would find other paediatric anaesthesiologists to take my place because I planned to leave. Understandably, he was totally disbelieving and astonished. But at that moment I realized that fate engineered my exit. Life had finally made the decision inevitable for me ending my dithering of the past 18 months. I also understood that it is the 'blows' or downsides in life's journey that propel us to more purposeful trajectories in the future.

The next morning, I experienced an indescribable feeling of profound peace as I woke up. I said to Vasu, "Okay, not only do you have to support an unemployed wife, but also finance a budding pain specialist "wandering" about in the pain clinics abroad!" His response was characteristically, "Thank God that you have seen the light at last! Go wherever you want! Spend whatever you want but *please start!*" There is no way I can express what I felt at this great gift of confidence, support, and love that freed me to pursue whatever I wanted!

The next phase was sitting at home pouring over pain management tomes day-after-day studying far more than I did for my undergraduate or postgraduate studies. The 'pain' textbooks provided a tremendous amount of theoretical information but no specific instructions of what to do, when, or how, to relieve a particular pain. This was less than encouraging, but I doggedly kept going. At about the same time my son, Ananth, suffered a heavy-weightlifting injury. All the consultants, orthopaedic surgeons, sports medicine people, and physiotherapists could not really help him. That was when I realized how dire and unmet was the need for a pain specialist. Chronic pain was indeed a grey area for all doctors. Meanwhile, Ananth had immense pain, limping all the time, unable to attend college. In desperation I suggested acupuncture. Ananth agreed on the condition that I would do it. I had no knowledge or experience of acupuncture, but I requested Dr Yamuna, an anaesthesiologist who practiced it, to guide me. Slowly and gradually, Ananth improved even with my amateur foray into acupuncture. I was intrigued by this positive outcome and decided to learn acupuncture from Dr Anton Jayasuriya, a great teacher in Colombo, Sri Lanka, who had learnt acupuncture in China. Working with the supremely confident professor was a fascinating experience because he imbued his students and patients with the same. It was a revelation to see him nonchalantly treat, serious addictions, medical, and neurological conditions. It was an interesting experience to be focused fulltime on acupuncture for one month, at a distance from all my knowledge of allopathy. It also confirmed certain thoughts of mine, why allopathy, which is all of 200 years old is called "mainstream" medicine, while all other systems like Ayurveda, traditional Chinese medicine, naturopathy, among others, with a documented history of thousands of years are 'alternative' medicine. I had always wondered, 'alternative' to what? Obviously to 'mainstream' allopathy. This anachronism is perhaps the child of British colonialization, which made English a 'global' language. A wise person once commented that science is all about hypotheses, which are all about the opinions of one who talks loudest and longest. Therefore, only those who can publish in English can be mainstream. Anything which is not taught or published in English is 'alternative'.

However, I found that although acupuncture provided good answers to many medical conditions, it was rather vague about chronic pains. The concepts of acupuncture were quite similar to Ayurveda with a lot of metaphysical content, which was so different to allopathy that my brain became a zone of conflict between the two diametrically opposite ideologies. I felt it was better for me to enhance my core strength and pursue pain management from an allopathic perspective since there was a lot of new pain research in the USA and UK. Thus, I returned to India, armed with an introduction to acupuncture but with the clear understanding that I would use it only to augment my allopathic approach to pain management.

For the next phase in my education, I had to visit some modern pain clinics abroad to understand the technology to treat pain, since there were no dedicated, fulltime pain clinics in India at that time. I wrote to some of my anaesthesia colleagues from the USA and the UK, Singapore, and Japan to organize an observer's post in the pain clinics there. That was when I realized that in other countries also, people were not very aware of pain management. But my friends helped with introductions to pain specialists in these countries and I spent the next several months visiting these places.

The journey continued, but now with a clear focus and finally, on November 27, 2005, Ashirvad, the blessing, became a reality.

Introduction

Pain, the oldest symptom of human suffering, has given birth to several systems of medicine. Protracted and severe pain strikes at the root of the personality taking away self-respect, self-confidence, and personal, financial, and emotional independence. Albert Schweitzer declared, "Pain is a more terrible lord of mankind than even death itself." To establish pain management as a new specialty, pioneering work was done by John Joseph Bonica, Rene Leriche, Jonas Henrik Kellgren, Chit Chan Gunn, Janet G. Travell, and David G. Simmons. Braving criticism of colleagues and peers, they documented chronic pain conditions to open the doors to a new specialty. Schweitzer's words, "We must all die, but that I can spare him suffering, that, is my ever-new privilege," resonate everyday at Ashirvad.

Contemporary pain management comprises some very sophisticated treatments, addressing various parts of the nervous system that are historically assumed to be responsible for pain. Yet, neuropathic pains remain untreatable enigmas. Opioids are generously prescribed to cover the residual pains persisting after neural interventions, culminating in an opioid crisis in the US.

Over the past several years, working with pain management, I have understood and realized that novel concepts, which look at pain generators from new perspectives, are necessary to develop innovations. Like a physician of ancient times, I have observed my patients, listened to their stories, evolved the concept that all neuropathies (nerve lesions) are actually neuromyopathies (diseases of nerves *and* muscles) giving rise to the ubiquitously present myofascial pains. My new system of pain management is gratifyingly effective in curing common and uncommon conditions, considered to be extremely difficult, including Complex Regional Pain Syndrome (CRPS), chronic pelvic pains, chronic orofacial pains, neuropathic pains of all varieties including post-surgical pains, failed back surgery pains, and cancer pains. I have done this simply by considering all chronic pains to be neuromyopathic with a major muscle-pain component including common problems like frozen shoulder, osteoarthritis, rheumatoid arthritis, spondylitis, and backache.

The field of pain management

During my visits abroad, figuring out the feasibility of establishing a pain clinic, given the myriad infrastructural problems in India, I gathered the following impressions.

Well-equipped: The US and UK pain clinics were very well equipped, staffed, and organized. I particularly liked the doctor-patient interactions at Bradford, UK where my friend Sanjeeva Gupta graciously organized an observer's post for me. I realized that this sophisticated level of establishment would only be possible if I did it myself, at my cost. No Indian institution or hospital, public or private sector, would readily make a heavy financial investment on a hitherto unknown specialty, to establish a state-of-the-art pain clinic in India.

Back pain dominates: I visited four major centres in the USA, two in the UK, and one each in Singapore and Japan. Everywhere, overwhelmingly and repeatedly back pain dominated the pain type. Thus, I decided that my first priority would be to learn the intricacies of spinal pain from a spine surgeon.

Understanding pain: After a year of gruelling study of contemporary pain literature and pain management at pain clinics, I felt confident to actually take on the challenge of understanding chronic pain. While I was not any wiser, at least I knew what the experts around the world thought, taught, and how they addressed several pain conditions. One major factor that enhanced my understanding was my personal experience of various chronic pains such as mechanical backache, cervical spondylitis, migraine, herpes zoster pain, and subsequent postherpetic neuralgia (PHN). I have gone through 'natural' labour pains thrice without pain killers because I wanted to understand the nature of pain. Therefore, I knew what acute and chronic pain felt like.

The realization dawned upon me that the advanced treatments carried out in sophisticated centers in the west were equally feasible every where Although the necessary equipments were available, assembling them would take time, effort, and a huge investment. Dr Shailen Jalali at the Jefferson pain clinic, Philadelphia, advised me to develop a patient-base by working in some hospitals, to establish a practice and make myself visible. This would ensure that when the pain clinic was indeed set up, it would have a better chance of breaking even, because some awareness and credibility would have been already established. This was valuable and sound advice, although I had initial doubts about whether hospitals in Mumbai would have the vision to provide the necessary space and time to establish a pain clinic.

Back in Mumbai, I learnt about back and other orthopaedic pains from Dr Ingalhalikar, an excellent spine surgeon who had the foresight to appreciate that nonsurgical management of back pain was essential to avoid back surgery. In the 1990s, he had established a patient-education endeavour called, "Back School" to educate patients about back pain in Thane, a Mumbai suburb. A generous teacher, he taught me the art of examining and interpreting symptoms, and treatment of not just back pain but other types of locomotor pains (knee, shoulder, and hip, among others) from the orthopaedic perspective. More importantly, he taught me the finer nuances of caring between a doctor and a pain patient. I also attended the MRI centre at Jaslok Hospital to understand the information from MRIs in various pain conditions, particularly spine pains.

My scepticism about hospitals supporting a new specialty was justified. I wrote to six public and private hospitals, none responded. The authorities at All-India Institute of Physical Medicine and Rehabilitation (AIIPMR), where I had rendered honorary service for a year, wanted me to work unofficially and honorarily. After a lifetime of rendering free work in general hospitals, I had realized that it has no value nor credibility. The unofficial pain clinic would be at the mercy of the administration and could be shut down at any time. Therefore, I regretfully declined the offer despite the attraction of AIIPMR as a centrally-funded rehabilitation centre with all infrastructure essential for a pain clinic including an operation theatre, physiotherapy and psychotherapy departments. Therefore, it became increasingly evident that if a pain clinic had to be established in Mumbai, I would have to undertake the task myself.

At this juncture, the ideal break came as advice from my friend and mentor, Dr Meher Elavia, the CEO of Prince Alykhan Hospital (PAKH) in Mazgaon, to establish a pain clinic at PAKH before starting out independently. Thus in 2003, the pain clinic was established with her support and considerable goodwill. This hospital was a boon to my fledgling practice because Dr Pradhan, the cancer surgeon, and Dr Kapadia the orthopaedic surgeon, gave unstinting support by referring pain patients to me. At our very first meeting Dr MA Khan the neurologist promised me that he would ensure that the pain clinic would get enough patients. This was a great help because I could prove that pain deserved proper attention and treatment. Within three months at PAKH, I treated several varieties of pain and the need for a pain clinic was unequivocally vindicated. Attendance at the pain clinic quadrupled and I did the ultimate procedure in pain management, intrathecal pump implantation. This was the first such procedure in western India. Until then, it was done only at the All-India Institute of Medical Sciences (AIIMS) in Delhi.

This case made most of the consultants sit up and take notice because the patient had been in and out of PAKH for several years with health issues including excruciating pain from failed back surgery. They were amazed to see her pain-free, happily going about her life in a manner hitherto unimaginable. It also dispelled the subtle unacknowledged myth in most medical minds that pain is more "in the head".

Additionally, I began working at the Breach Candy Hospital and engaged in discussions with Dr Krishna Joshi, my mentor from my years in anaesthesia, regarding the possibility of establishing a private clinic. He has always given me sound advice, encouragement, and unstinting help. I diligently followed his advice, "Focus on building a good reputation, and lucrative practice will follow." When I went to meet Dr Joshi, Dr Laud, a senior orthopaedic surgeon who was with him, advised that I should start a clinic in Dadar, a central Mumbai location. He stressed the need to be around senior consultants who understood the difficulty of treating chronic pain and that he would refer his pain patients to me. This was a very unexpected but welcome development. True to his word, he sent me two patients on the very first day of my practice and has supported me since. Patients play a vital role in any doctor's practice as they provide opportunities for doctors to demonstrate their skills and expertise. I was extremely fortunate to have the trust of senior consultants and unconditional wholehearted support of anaesthesiologists who are highly respected and influential members within the medical profession. My anaesthesiology network was huge because of my paediatric anaesthesia teaching activities, and this brought referrals from orthopaedics, surgeons, neurosurgeons, and many others whom I had never even met. Thus, a full-fledged pain management practice, which keep me busy throughout the day, took off with minimal effort.

Private practice in pain management

I was the first fulltime pain specialist to establish a day-care centre in Mumbai, dedicated exclusively to the treatment of chronic pain, unattached to any corporate set up. That gave impetus to my practice.

Initial hiccups: A disconcerting discovery, however, was that after initial pain relief (sometimes spectacular relief) with interventional pain procedures, patients kept returning with pain recurrence. I was unhappy, to say the least, but I could not fathom why the pain returned despite me doing everything correctly with textbook precision. All my professional life I had worked in some honorary capacity and the preceding two years had been entirely pro bono work. And now, experiencing unsatisfactory outcomes despite providing expensive treatments made me feel inadequate. Had I been my patient, I would certainly not have been happy! I seriously considered that if this was the extent of my efficacy as a pain specialist, then I should retire!

A timely eye opener: Three months into my practice, I met Dr. Chan Gunn an authority on myofascial pain syndromes (MPS) in Bangkok, when he came up to complement me on the practical utility of my talk on paediatric regional anaesthesia. I was delighted and said that I was honoured to meet him, having read his important and extremely interesting chapter on MPS in Bonica's *Management of Pain* (a pain specialist's bible). Very graciously, he invited me to attend his MPS workshop the next day although it was over booked.

The workshop was an eye-opener as it introduced me to a very important perspective, on the major role of muscles in pain. But for the small chapter in Bonica's textbook, there was hardly any literature on muscle pains while there were many books on nerves and nerve blocks, with details of why, where, when, and how to administer them, their probable benefits, and so on. None of these books mentioned muscle pain except in passing, as a lip service. Dr Gunn had a completely different perspective that many pains could be entirely or primarily due to the muscles, and these could be relieved by a definite treatment called intramuscular stimulation (IMS) where very fine acupuncture needles are inserted into the muscles

Table 1. The difference between acupuncture and IMS as per Dr Chan Gunn.[1]

Parameter	Dry needling	Acupuncture
Thickness of needles	30–34-gauge solid needles	30–34-gauge solid needles
Needle length	13–50 mm long	13–25 mm long
Target	The needle is inserted into a painful point anywhere in an anatomically defined muscle. Allopathy, anatomy have no concept of meridians.	Accurately defined acupoints located on energy channels (meridians). Acupuncture has no concept of muscles.
Diagnosis	Requires specialized examination to detect tender points, a jump sign, and a palpable taut band in the muscle.	Based on history of illness, pulse diagnosis, and metaphysical theories that link the meridians to symptoms.
Mode of action	The needle entry into the muscle causes stimulation to make it jump and hence the name intramuscular stimulation (IMS)	Needle entry into the energy channel is either to let out the excess of energy or add extra energy to improve energy flow.
Local twitch reflex (LTR)	LTR is an involuntary muscle twitch at a myofascial trigger point (MTrP) when a needle is introduced, moved around, and pumped quickly.	No attempt is made to elicit a LTR since there is no concept of MTrP in acupuncture.
Target tissues	Intramuscular stimulation/DN deals with abnormality in the muscle that causes pain.	Acupuncture only addresses the disordered energy flow in disease.
Target disease	DN or IMS is developed to address myofascial pain and relaxation of taut bands in MPS.	Acupuncture addressed many diseases and not just chronic pain.
Difference in structural concepts	The MTrPs are located inside the muscle and knowledge of muscle anatomy is essential.	The anatomically indemonstrable meridians are dedicated to the heart, lung, pericardium, liver, gall bladder urinary bladder, small and large intestines, and even to anatomically non-existent structures called the triple warmer, Du and Ren meridians.

(Table 1). However, IMS is not acupuncture and since there is no injection involved it is also called dry needling (DN).

Moving forward

After returning from Bangkok, I started using IMS/DN on patients who had recurrent pain after interventional pain procedures, where I suspected MPS. My acupuncture training made it easy for me to master the technique, which differed from the Gunn technique of IMS from the very beginning. I used more needles, and I followed the acupuncture principle of leaving the needles in for 20 minutes to get the maximum effect after subjecting the patient to needle pain. This proved scientifically fortuitous since I discovered later with ultrasound visualization, that it takes 20–30 minutes for the needles to exert their effect. Therefore, my initial needling techniques incorporated both principles: it addressed muscles, unlike acupuncture, but the needles stayed in for longer, unlike worldwide DN techniques.

Very soon, I found that the pain relief was not just consistent but astonishing in all pains; particularly, those persisting after blocks. Lackadaisical as it was, my DN still succeeded in reversing many pain conditions, which were not considered to be myofascial at all, like frank neuropathic pains, discogenic back pain, carpal tunnel syndrome, and trigger finger among others. Along with pain relief, patients seemed to have improved activity levels.

Even some bedridden patients improved after DN! One patient, from Rajasthan, was brought on a stretcher with a urinary catheter, because he was paralysed. I treated him with an epidural steroid injection, which relieved his pain but not his paralysis. But with dry needling, he slowly improved, started walking with crutches and after an uneventful catheter removal, was discharged. Imagine my astonishment a year later, when a patient's husband smiled and asked me, "Doctor, you did not recognize me?" For the life of me I could not place him, but he triumphantly told me that he was my erstwhile paralysed patient who had completely recovered! I could not believe him because at that stage of my practice my understanding of muscle pathology was rudimentary, and I had little idea of the power of dry needling. So, I asked him repeatedly for all the details, which he clarified. He gleefully told me that he had travelled by train from Rajasthan, carried all the luggage himself while also assisting his wife. Thereafter, every now and then he would bring patients from his village for treatment. By now, I realized that I was onto something very significant, almost spectacular! My practice, which had been ordinary and quasi-successful before the introduction of IMS/DN in my treatments, had now become fascinating because of the newfound, but largely unexplained success with DN.

The big step towards pain management

In 2004, I bought a place in Hindu Colony of Dadar. Finally, I could set up a pain clinic as I wanted to, similar to pain clinics in the USA! However, after a lifetime of working in an honorary capacity in public hospitals, I had no savings or capital to fall back on. My greatest strength was that I had Vasu, as my guarantor.

This truth was brought home to me in unvarnished starkness when I applied for a bank loan. Both the bank manager and the loan consultant looked askance at my non-existent income of the previous two years and asked me point blank how I hoped to repay their loan even if they decided to sanction it! Nobody like a banker to bring one down to earth! My explanations of a sabbatical year for study, and unpaid honorary work at AIIPMR before that, sounded utterly feeble, even to my own ears. Talk about being cut down to size! As usual, I turned to Vasu to get me out of the *impasse*. And, as always, he took charge. I don't know what he did to convince the bankers, but convince them, he did. Ashirvad Pain Relief Clinic was inaugurated on November 27, 2005, by my revered teacher, Dr YG Bhojraj, who had been my mentor in the ups and downs of my professional career.

Reinventing myself: I decided to return to the anatomy cadaver lab to relearn muscle anatomy to improve my DN technique, which was still rudimentary. It came as a rude awakening that after 15 days, I had not even begun to understand the basics of muscle anatomy!

Rakhi More, the anatomy lecturer assigned to me, assuaged my dismay by explaining that the undergraduate curriculum does not include detailed muscle anatomy courses. Eventually, it took me six months of daily dissection to get a working idea of muscle anatomy. With this newly acquired knowledge, I refined the DN techniques tremendously and transformed it into the ultrasound guided dry needling (USGDN) that we practice today. Application of this refined technique to various pains and correlating it to patients' feedback opened up new avenues of thought on several conditions and helped to develop many out-of-the-box ideas that gave rise to a completely new understanding of pain. My patients became my teachers, teaching me on the job that there is hardly any pain that does not have an acceptable cure or management. This book is about this journey of discovery as I relive the learning experiences from one patient to the next.

Reference

[1] Gunn, C.C. and P.D. Wall. 1996. The Gunn Approach to the Treatment of Chronic Pain: Intramuscular Stimulation for Myofascial Pain of Radiculopathic Origin. Churchill Livingstone, London.

Chapter 1

Understanding the Concept of Pain

Etymology of Pain: Middle English, from Anglo-French *peine* (pain, suffering), from Latin *poena* (penalty, punishment), from Greek *poine* (payment, penalty, recompense).

What is pain?

Pain is a sensation that the body uses to sound an alert to bodily injury. Cuts, crushes, burns, surgery, illness, blood supply reduction, inflammation, or anything that damages tissues will cause pain. Individuals understand pain through experience. The inability to communicate does not mean the absence of pain. The dictum in pain management according to pain nurse, Margo McCaffery (1968)[1] is, "Pain is whatever the experiencing patient says is existing, whenever he/she says it does." Patients describe sensations of aching, pulling, tearing, tingling, electrical shocks, burning, insect crawling, or ants biting, to name a few, even when there is no obvious injury on the body nor are ants or insects inside. Hence The International Association for the Study of Pain (IASP) defines pain[2] as, "An unpleasant sensory and emotional experience associated with or resembling that associated with actual or potential tissue damage."

Pain is a subjective experience that is influenced to varying degrees by biological (body), psychological (mind), and social factors, hence it is called a biopsychosocial phenomenon. Physical pain is a sensation

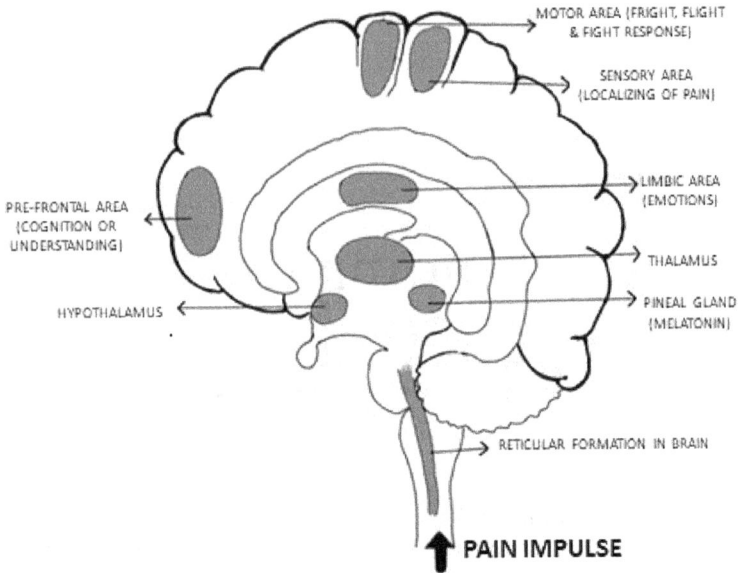

Figure 2. Functional magnetic resonance imaging (fmri) details complexity of current pain perception.

while the total experience of pain is a combination of physical pain as interpreted by the mind. The thalamus, a centre in the lower part of the brain, perceives the *sensation* of pain. Multiple locations of the cerebral cortex get involved in the *experience* of pain, as seen in fMRI studies of the brain (Figure 2).

Mechanism of pain perception: From physical injury to pain sensation

Pain sensation begins with specialized miniature organs called nociceptors (receptors designed to detect pain) or free nerve endings in the skin and various other tissues. Nature has placed millions of nociceptors in the skin, joints, muscles, and connective tissues, as well as in the protective membranes around our internal organs and bones to sense any stimulus that can cause bodily harm. Nociceptors are connected to the thinnest of nerve fibres called the C fibres and the slightly thicker A delta fibres with a covering called the myelin sheath.

Types of nociceptors:

- *Mechanoreceptors* respond to high intensity mechanical stimuli such as a slap, a smash from a hammer, painful joint movements, distension of the hollow intestines, or stretching of the capsule of solid organs like the liver and kidney.
- *Thermal receptors* respond to temperature, such as the touch of a hot plate, warm bath, or freezing water.
- *Chemoreceptors* are present in the skin, muscles, nerves, connective tissues, joints, and the gut to sense the chemicals released by the huge chemical factory, the human body, in response to injury, infection, and inflammation. They also sense external toxic or hazardous chemicals.
- *Polymodal receptors* are free nerve endings that can assume the role of any receptor. Free nerve endings are called "silent receptors" since they *only* become active when they get sensitized over time, to respond to pain from various high-intensity thermal (< 10°C and > 40°C) and mechanical stimuli. Muscles have multitudes of polymodal receptors, which makes pain a very significant muscle sensation.

The receptors endow an evolutionary capability that allows differentiation between a pleasant touch, a painless touch, pressure of a powerful grip, and a painful grip. Thermal receptors not only help to avoid damage from extreme temperatures but also to automatically sense and maintain an optimal body temperature.

Injurious stimuli activate nociceptors, which send electrical impulses, via the nerves, to the spinal cord and then along a specialized pain pathway, which terminates in the thalamus and thereafter in the brain.

The relationship between pain and injury; Exploring the connection

A trivial injury can result in severe pain and contrarily, a severe injury may not always cause too much pain because the signal of an injury travelling up the anatomical pain pathway to the brain is subject to modulation to become a biopsychosocial phenomenon.

- *Biological*: Tissue damage in acute pain is obvious but in chronic pain, the tissue injury may not be discernible on the outside but could be real enough for the muscle nociceptors to convey an unpleasant sensation to the brain as is explained in later chapters.

- *Psychological*: The emotional (also called affective) aspect of pain is much more complex. One understands the pain sensation only when experiencing it. Nature makes sure that one avoids dangerous activities by making pain unpleasant so that pain is never ignored. If there was no experience of pain, people would try foolhardy antics, like sticking a hand in fire, jumping off the roof, crashing a hammer on the hand, or whatever took their fancy. The unpleasantness of the emotional experience induces a fear of pain, which makes one wary and careful in daily actions. The first experience of pain is usually in childhood, related to some injury such as a fall, vaccination, an injection, or a stomach ache. A personalized concept of pain based on the learning and understanding of its unpleasantness is thus formed in the mind and through life's experiences, subjective and psychological conclusions are drawn of what causes pain and how.

- *Social*: If society frowns upon loud exhibition of pain, people learn to avoid reacting loudly. But if society has no such norms the tendency would, more likely, be to highlight the pain rather than curtail it. By a process of constant learning in a social and cultural perspective, individual behaviour gets modelled by societal norms.

Understanding the pain pathway; Exploring how pain signals are transmitted

The afferent nerve from the pain-sensing nociceptor in the body surface up to the spinal cord represents the long tail called axon of the first-order neuron, which has its main cell body in the spinal cord. The nociceptor, the afferent nerve, and its cell body in the spinal cord, form the peripheral nervous system (PNS). The nerve from the spinal cord through the medulla oblongata, Pons, Midbrain, and thalamus right up to the cerebral cortex forms the second-order neuron belonging to the central nervous system (CNS). There might be a small interneuron interposed after the first neuron creating a third-order neuron (Figure 3). From the first-order neuron cell body at each spinal level, several branches emerge to form interconnections between the neighbouring first-, second-, and third-order neurons in the spinal segmental levels above and below, forming a complex neural network. These interconnections are pain

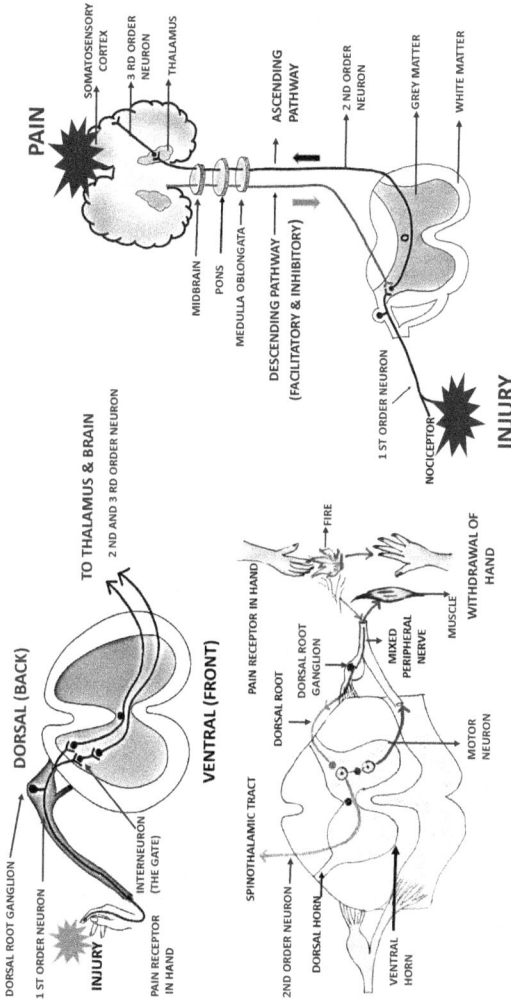

Figure 3. Top Left : Pain impulses from periphery travel in the first order neuron to spinal cord. The 2nd and 3rd order neurones carry the impulses onwards. Bottom Left : Pain impulses from a hand injury travel to the spinal cord, connect through interneurons to the motor nerves at the same level, to perform the "withdrawal reflex" at the spinal level, without conscious awareness. Right: Pain travels up the pain pathway to the thalamus. Descending impulses from the brain can facilitate or inhibit pain transmission at the spinal cord.

modulation mechanisms designed with the capability to increase or decrease the excitability and transmission in the pain pathway.

The connection between two neurons is through a gap, the synapse. When the electrical impulse in the nerve reaches its terminal at the synapse, it discharges chemicals called neurotransmitters, whose molecules bridge the gap between the two neurons and generate a similar electrical impulse in the next neuron (second- and third-order neurons) that moves along the pain pathway to the final terminus for physical pain, the thalamus. Perceptions and transmission of all sensations are mediated by these electrochemical interactions not just for pain but for every neural activity. The mind and ego, which together define the personality, the character, intelligence, and integrity of an individual—all these personality attributes are outcome of the sum total of the electrochemical activities in the brain. Additionally, these determine happiness, peace, bliss, ecstasy, valour, anger, resentment, anxiety, sorrow, depression, fear, and helplessness. These electrochemical interactions can be modified by medications called *neuromodulators*. These are not painkillers (which are usually anti-inflammatories or opioids) but they reduce pain significantly by altering the impulse traffic in the pain pathway. They also have a calming effect on the mind, may induce sleep, and reduce anxiety and depression. The primary purpose in using these drugs, however, is to alleviate pain; any benefit on the mind is an incidental bonus.

At the thalamus, pain is perceived as a vague, ill-defined sensation. Nature has provided an inbuilt neural pathway called thalamic projections, which emanate from the thalamus to various parts of the brain to culminate in the enigma of the sensation generically referred to as pain and suffering.

The transformation of a physical sensation into pain and suffering: Exploring the mechanisms and factors involved

The pain sensation at the thalamus becomes an accurate sensation by virtue of neural projections which reach various parts of the brain (Figure 4).

Sensory cortex: Thalamic projections travel accurately to the part of the cerebral cortex designated to receive physical sensations of a specific body part to register the pain intensity, location, and nature. For instance, one can localize a pinprick to the inside of the little finger because the

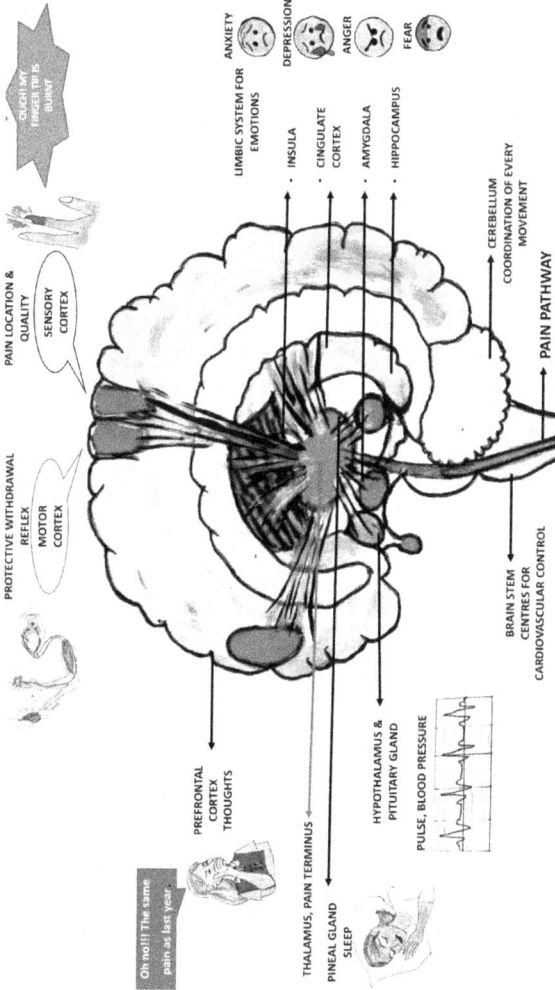

Figure 4. The pain impulses terminate at the thalamus. Thalamic projections to sensory, motor, cognitive (thought), and emotional centres define the complex unpleasant pain sensation. For eg the projection to the frontal cortex identifies the pain as the same burning pain in the tip of the same finger as the one experienced the previous year.

projections travel exactly to the area designated to receive the little finger sensations.

Motor cortex: Projections to the cerebral cortex responsible for movements initiate a protective limb withdrawal from the cause of pain. The withdrawal reflex occurs at the spinal cord (Figure 3) like snatching the hand off a hotplate in a split second. An automatic stiffening of the muscles around an injured area is nature's way of 'splinting' the area to avoid further damage or pain. For example, holding the fractured limb immobile or stiffening the abdominal wall in appendicitis.

Frontal cortex: The frontal cortex draws conclusions about the nature of pain, how it must have happened? Has one experienced a similar pain before, or is it unknown? Is the pain bearable or unbearable? Why is it so intense? Which part of the body has the pain? What can be done about it and how it could have been avoided? Projections to this part of the brain, concerned with cognition and intellect, help to formulate an intelligent and logical understanding of the pain.

Autonomic centres in the brain: Thalamic projections also reach these areas to increase the heart rate and blood pressure necessary for escaping/fleeing from the emergency situation causing pain. Thus, severe pain can initiate the flight, fight, or flight reflex (also called the stress response).

Sleep centres: Thalamic projections to brain areas initiating and maintaining sleep link pain with sleep disturbances.

Limbic cortex, amygdala, and insula: The most important projection goes to the limbic system responsible for producing the emotional responses of distress, fear, and danger, associated with pain. Thalamic projections to these areas lead to associated emotions like fear, anger, resentment, anxiety, and depression to make unpleasantness an invariable aspect of pain.

To summarize, projections to cortical areas transform the vague physical pain sensation at the thalamus to a specific precisely-located sensation, which evokes built-in protective automatic responses. The projections to the emotion centres make pain a complex perception that influences thoughts, ideas, and emotions, which make pain unpleasant, unwanted, and absolutely to be avoided. Conversely, the gamut of negative thoughts and decisions generated by our intellect and emotions, such as fear, anxiety, depression, mood swings, can exacerbate pre-existing pain, making pain and emotion/cognition a two-way street. All mental activities can magnify the quality and intensity of pain perception. It is this interdependence and interconnectivity between the mind and pain that makes it such a personal experience and a very flummoxing problem to solve.

The combination of the sensory, motor, cognitive, and emotional experiences of pain can trigger a simple withdrawal of the hand or a much more complex fright/flight/fight reflex designed by nature to protect the primitive man from danger, fleeing from the heat of a forest fire or from the fear of a snake. Unfortunately, chronic pain is not something one can flee from, yet the stressful emotional responses of danger, fear, anger, aversion, resentment, helplessness, anxiety, and depression continue unabated. Therefore, pain management has to use a holistic psychophysical approach that addresses not only the nerves carrying 'pain' to the thalamus and beyond, but also the mind that transforms physical pain into mental suffering.

The protective nature of pain: Examining its role and exceptions

Pain is one of the body's most important communication tools to warn that something is wrong and needs urgent attention. Without pain, bodies would be destroyed long before reaching teenage as it happens with some children who are born with a congenital 'absence' of pain. They lack the sodium channels in the nerves that initiate the electrochemical reactions to convey pain. Such children don't develop the protective mechanisms that make them fear or avoid noxious stimuli and because of repeated and severe injuries, they seldom live beyond the first two decades of life. Imagine, for instance, what would happen if one felt nothing when touching a hot stove or smashing a hammer on the hand.

Pain serves the vital function of protecting the body's integrity and as such nature has placed many failsafe mechanisms to ensure that pain *is always* felt, and protective action can be initiated immediately. This works well in acute pain, which protects by ensuring that one runs from danger or seeks immediate medical attention. But in chronic pain, the same mechanisms assume ominous overtones; the inbuilt protective mechanisms stay in overdrive, making it impossible to ignore the pain. The pain sensation goes rogue, ensuring that the pain itself becomes the disease.

Understanding chronic pain: Mechanisms, impact and treatment

Peripheral sensitization: In addition to the nociceptors, which automatically respond to injury, many additional, but normally inactive, 'silent' or 'sleeping' multipotent (polymodal) free nerve endings develop spontaneous activity when the injury continues, or when inflammation ensues secondary to injury. Pain from a cut or an abrasion may initially be intense but it acquires a much more unpleasant quality and intensity later as inflammation sets in to make the wound hot, red, and swollen. This happens with all injuries. In addition to recruiting the sleeping receptors, the chemicals released by inflammation also increase the number of impulses, their frequency and intensity in the afferent pain-carrying nerves all along the pain pathway, right up to the thalamus. The excitement in afferent nerves up to the spinal cord is collectively called peripheral sensitization (Figure 5). The muscle has an abundance of polymodal receptors coupled with the innate capability to generate an inflammatory response thereby ensuring that muscle pain is never ignored.

Central sensitization: The pain pathway is not a passive, static, bundle of nerves that just carries the electrical impulses of pain sensation but it is a functionally dynamic system that is subject to constant modification (modulation) by its network of interconnections (Figure 3). All along the pain pathway, from the spinal cord up to the brain, nerves keep communicating with their counterparts from other levels. This mind boggling multitude of interconnections within the CNS, become hyperactive when pain becomes chronic. The constant traffic of impulses in the pain pathway in persistent or chronic pain causes a state of hyperactivity in all the interconnections that connect the pain pathway to myriad other parts of the nervous system (central sensitization). This state of global hyperactivity in the pain pathway and rest of the nervous system has the potential to become autonomous (independent of the original pain) and sustain itself in chronic pain states. The influences from these interconnections in the pain pathway have the capacity to multiply pain several times (Figure 6). Decisive control of pain with an intervention (complete pain relief, a total holiday from pain) even for a day, could reduce/stop this hyperactivity to make a major difference to chronic pain patients (Figures 6, 7) Neuromodulator medications,

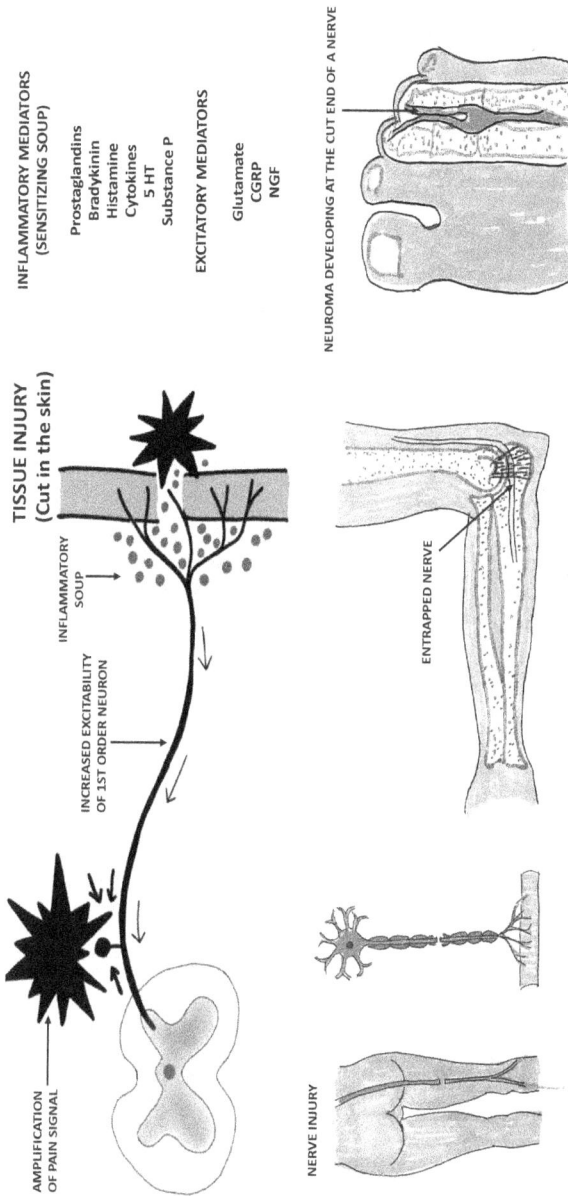

Figure 5. Top: Injury causes inflammatory response, increasing the uptake and traffic of electrical impulses in PNS, resulting in peripheral sensitization with pain amplification. Bottom: Forms of nerve injury–cuts, compression against bones, and a neuroma cause neuropathic pains.

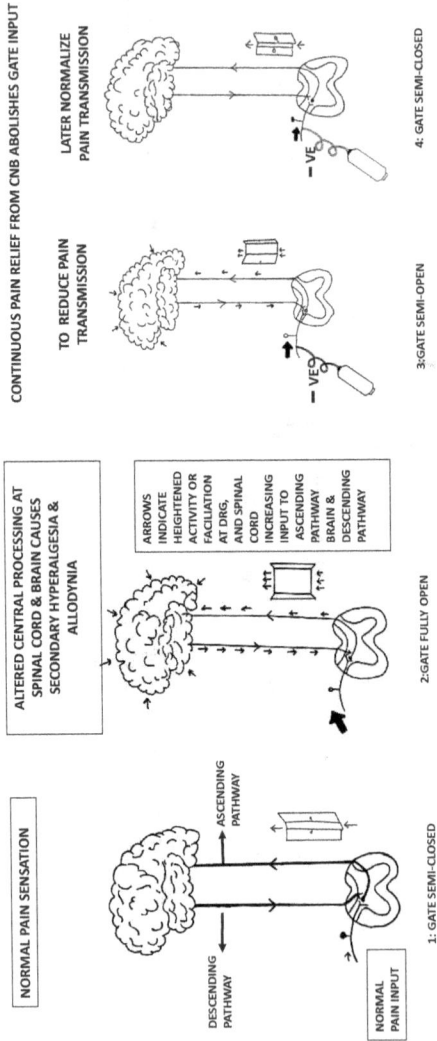

Figure 6. The normal pain pathway (sparse arrows). 2: Increased pain traffic (more arrows) and open gate increasing pain sensitivity (secondary hyperalgesia and allodynia). 3: Partial gate closure after two weeks of continuous nerve block (CNB) with unwinding (gate semi-open). 4: Normal traffic after complete unwinding.

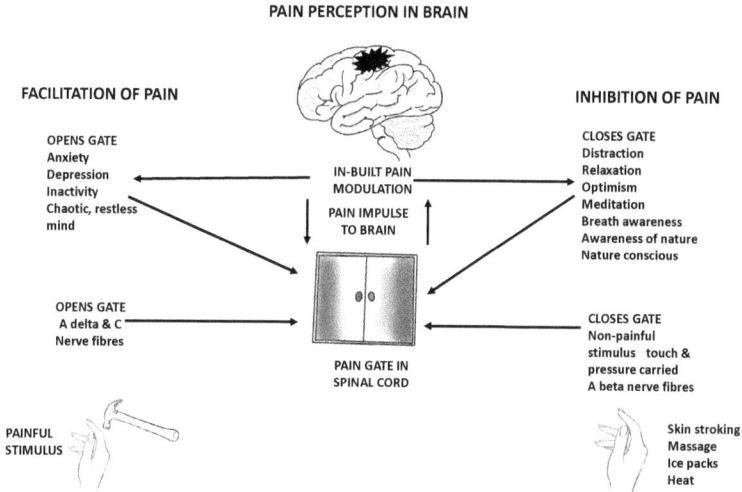

Figure 7. The spinal cord neural gate blocks mild pains, allows persistent higher intensity pains through to allow pain perception and swift protective action. Emotions also influence the gate.

mindfulness, meditation, and similar techniques can also attenuate pain, albeit to a much lesser extent than our powerful interventional treatments.

Variability in the experience of pain

Pain is a highly personalized sensation and people respond to it in many ways. The pain that one person can ignore might be incapacitating to another person because pain perception involves not only the body but also the mind, moods, and life situations forming a complex mosaic of psychological, emotional, and social influences.

How we feel pain and how we react to it depends not only on the cause, but also on personal, genetic, individual and emotional traits superimposed on a backdrop of ethnic, social influences and cultural beliefs with which we grow up. These determine the structural configuration of the pain centres in the brain; response to pain is heavily influenced by the momentary emotional aberrations, past learning experiences, pain memories not just in the physical pain pathways but also in the emotional centres of the brain. All these factors together create different levels of tolerance or sensitivity to pain and our consequent response.

Genetics

The genetic makeup determines how the interconnections in the pain pathway can facilitate transmission by lowering thresholds to pain transmission to the brain and/or interfere with the built-in pain inhibition mechanisms. The electrochemical activities, which determine how pain is processed in the pain pathway are influenced by the sodium, calcium, and potassium ion channels in the nerves and the presence, relative excesses or paucity/absences of the chemicals called neurotransmitters.

Evidence suggests that genetic factors may influence the tendency to develop chronic pains after even a trivial injury, be more receptive to pain, or develop neuropathic pain after a nerve injury. It is important to understand how different organs in the body process the pain medications.

Ethnicity

Certain ethnic groups may have a similar genetic composition, which in turn determines many bodily functions. For example, absorption of vitamin B12 may be compromised in Indian vegetarians. The main source for vitamin B12 is meat eggs and milk and low values of vitamin B12 levels are routinely seen in vegetarian patients. However, low values are even seen in daily meat-eaters leading to the possibility that there might be ethnic groups among Indians who are prone to B12 deficiency (Ashirvad unpublished data). In contrast, the normal vitamin B12 values seen in vegetarians whose food contains no vitamin B12 may be because of gut microbial contribution. Vitamin deficiencies may have a role in the initial incidence of pain as well as in its recurrences after having been corrected. After corrective injections patients enjoy a few pain-free years after which pains recur consequent to consumption of the replenished vitamin stores for bodily functions in the interim period.

Case study: A young adult presented with carpal tunnel pain in the hand due to excessive computer usage. His vitamin deficiencies were corrected during treatment. Three years after recovering he came down with mechanical back pain. The MRI was normal but the vitamin B12 was a dismal 68 pg/ml (picograms per millilitre) as against the normal 190–950 pg/ml. This was probably the reason for the back sprain despite regular exercises. He responded to treatment of muscle sprain with ultrasound guided dry needling (USGDN). It was important to check the entire family (as they share similar genetics and diet). Although they were asymptomatic, all members showed abysmally low vitamin B12 levels and had to receive vitamin injections.

Cultural beliefs

Social and cultural learning impacts how patients describe their symptoms according to their worldview, which may be very different from a doctor's biomedical view with a specific vocabulary regarding diseases. Almost all theistic belief systems have the concepts of cause and effect, and physical suffering is often taken as a consequence of that.

Karma (an Indian/Hindu belief) implies that every action has an inexorable but logical consequence; that pain and suffering are a consequence for past actions, committed not just in this life but in previous lifetimes. This leads to a certain level of stoic acceptance of life's reverses, including pain and suffering, by those who acknowledge *karma* as a system of the even distribution of justice. This is more among the elderly who unequivocally believe in this concept and thus receive any pain relief with a lot of gratitude. The younger generation, with no such recourse of passing the buck onto *karma*, suffer more because they believe that the buck of their life stops with them. Not only do they have physical distress but are plagued by anxieties and resentments like, "*Why is this happening to me*? How can I be in pain at such a young age? Why am I experiencing this pain when I'm following all the advice from the Internet, Google and social media regarding proper eating, exercising and doing everything right?" Many patients automatically assume the worst from Internet medical information and go into a panic mode or anxiety and depression.

Case study: A young urology resident doctor was brought by his gynaecologist mother, for treatment of severe pain a year after herpes. As a doctor, he could understand medical jargon, and had read up everything about post-herpetic neuralgia (PHN), and despondently concluded that his condition was incurable and he had to live with it; worse still, he believed that this pain was associated with suicides, which had become his consideration in the worst-case scenario. Modern medicine has advanced so much that a specialist in one field knows precious little about other specialties, particularly chronic pain, which is not taught in the undergraduate or postgraduate curricula. He had neither seen chronic pain nor understood it so he was really a layperson in this field. He had ignored the positive treatments available but had focused on the worst aspect of postherpetic pain. He was so depressed that his worried mother, delegating her gynaecology practice to a deputy, was staying with him, to provide moral support. At the first consultation he categorically stated that he was resigned to lifelong pains that could lead to suicide. He was unconvinced by the scientific explanation about the cause of PHN and how PHN pain is routinely reversed so effectively with Ashirvad treatment that patients forget they ever had it. He agreed to the treatment more to appease his concerned mother than to any positive expectations from the treatment. A week after treatment he grudgingly admitted that he had 60 per cent pain relief but he also said, "The pain will surely come back." He had to be told sternly to listen to his body, which was telling him the pain was less and not to read anything further on this topic because he neither had the correct perspective nor the background experiential information. He was sent back to work and called at regular intervals for further treatment. After his third visit he had no pain but still feared its recurrence. Slowly, over the next few months, he realized that his pain was not recurring; he became more positive and his mother could return to her own life and work. This was the case with a medical doctor! One can only imagine what indiscriminate information from the Internet can do to laypersons, without the balancing filters of practical experience and expert discrimination to temper the information.

Gender

Women report more frequent, more severe, and longer-lasting pains than men. It's not known whether this is due to hormonal influences, biological differences, or psychological and social factors. In the mid-19th century Europe and America, hysteria and pain were widely diagnosed together in every community. The treatment was social isolation, confinement in bed, and exclusion from any form of intellectual activity, even sewing and reading. Invalids, mostly middle- and upper-class females filled homes, spas, and convalescent facilities. Fortunately, as opportunities for education improved, the disease called hysteria disappeared; virtually an eradication similar to that of yellow fever and influenza. Dr Doris Cope mentions in *Bonica's Management of Pain*[4] that in the 21st century fibromyalgia (FM) seems to be common in the affluent West while it is less reported in Asian and developing nations.

Other long-term health problems

Many chronic conditions, such as diabetes, FM, migraine headaches, and irritable bowel syndrome (IBS), are associated with pain.

Influence of gut microbiome in chronic pain: There are more microorganisms in the gut (called microbiome) and skin than the number of cells in the body. The microbiome includes bacteria, fungi, viruses, protozoa, and helminths, all forming a rich complex and ever-changing ecosystem. The microbiome composition is influenced by the person and environmental factors. The microbiome has effects on physiologic, metabolic, and immune functions of the host. These bi-directional effects may be caused by the infiltration of bacterial antigens eliciting an immune response in the host, secretion of biologically-active bacterial metabolites that affect multiple host organs, metabolism, and degradation of the food and medications ingested by the host, to name a few. One of the most interesting effects of gut microbiome is on the central nervous system (CNS). This so-called "gut-brain-axis" appears to be an intricate bi-directional communication between the gut and the brain, allowing members of the gut bacterial community to affect the function of the CNS nerve circuits. In recent years, there is a growing appreciation of the role of the gut and urine microbiome alterations as observed in IBS, chronic pelvic pain, chronic fatigue syndrome, FM, rheumatoid arthritis, ankylosing spondylitis, and Gulf-war syndrome; also, in gastrointestinal diseases, metabolic disorders, cardiovascular, skin, dental problems, and cancer.

Psychological factors

Johannes Peter Müller (1801–1858), stated in his book, *Handbuch der Physiologie des Menschen*[3] that "Pain is never a matter of sheer invention by the patient," yet a "stimulated imagination can increase existing pain and, in one so disposed, produce the pain that is sensed."

During the 18th–19th century the Western concept was that pain was majorly psychological and it was only after the American Civil War in 1865 and the World Wars that this concept changed. Inexplicable pains in young men could not be dismissed as merely psychological problems. Many empathetic physicians dedicated their lives to delve into the chronic pain mystery and their genuine interest and scientific enquiry led to the evolution of pain as a new specialty in the 1960s. The 1970s saw the emergence of the International Association for the Study of Pain, IASP with a dedicated research journal, *Pain*. The concept of interdisciplinary pain teams was initiated. Research into the various pain conditions led to a new understanding of pain mechanisms, its manifestations, development of medical and interventional treatments. Clinical diagnostic criteria were described for several conditions.

An exaggerated pessimism or 'catastrophizing' (imagining and fearing a catastrophe although nothing in the situation warrants it) of pain can also make it worse. There seems to be an association between the prevalence of pain and depression, anxiety, or low self-esteem. The absence of an objective measurement of pain, as with fever or blood pressure, complicates the "chicken and egg" situation between pain and emotions.

Social factors

Stress and social isolation worsen the pain experience. Research also suggests that poor education, low income, and unemployment are linked with a higher prevalence of pain. At Ashirvad, the importance of work is always emphasized and patients are strongly encouraged to return to work as soon as the pain becomes manageable.

Past experiences

Memories of past painful experiences can influence current experiences. If anyone has ever had a bad experience with a dentist or is very nervous without ever visiting a dentist, even a minor probe in the mouth can produce a strong pain response. Pain itself can predispose one to more pain. In fact, the most consistent risk factor for developing pain is a previous pain episode. Even infants and toddlers, who may not cry at the first or second vaccination will start crying the moment they enter the paediatrician's office in anticipation, recalling earlier painful experiences.

Other individual factors

General attitude, upbringing, strategies, and the ability to cope with stress can affect how pain messages are interpreted and to what degree the pain can be tolerated. Our preconceived notions or expectations as to how we think, or how we should feel or react, all reflect on the degree of pain.

Pain as a sensation to be learnt

Pain is a sensation that has to be learnt and the first introduction to it is, perhaps, in early childhood (1–9 years). A child does not understand the first experience of this new but very unpleasant sensation. It's frightening because it doesn't get wished away and worse still, the parents can't chase it away. This is probably the first time that a child realizes or senses that even parents can fail despite trying their best. This is even more frightening, and all that the hapless child knows is that there is no escape. This triggers the helpless and agitated screaming response, establishing the mental and emotionally fearful unpleasantness of the sensation, quite apart from the physical pain the child experiences. The sheer unpleasantness of pain etches the experience in the memory. However, if it is not a prolonged or chronic pain, the child won't remember it later. Most healthy children grow into adolescence (10–18 years) or adulthood without memories of personal pain.

Biological mechanisms for pain perception develop in mid- and late pregnancy when the baby is still in the mother' womb. Inbuilt capabilities to dampen or suppress pain mature later in infancy. Therefore, pre-term babies may be more susceptible to pain in the second and third trimesters of pregnancy. Most commonly, infants experience the first pain during immunizations. These are forgotten till they get some injury or experience pain due to some illness or injections. Traditionally, babies are closely nurtured and protected by adults and are rarely exposed to pain. However, technological advances in the care of pre-term new-borns have ensured the survival of medically fragile babies who spend weeks and months in the neonatal ICU, they undergo many painful procedures, surgery, and experience post-surgical pain but how much of it is remembered is not known. They certainly react to pain and often show an increase in pulse rate and blood pressure even to innocuous, daily routine care, like diaper changes. Dr Grunau and her team have, however, shown reassuring data from several countries that suggest that early-life pain does not predispose these babies to later life pain problems.[5]

Types of pain

Acute pain

Acute pain has a highly protective purpose and sounds alerts to injury thus protecting from further harm. It starts suddenly but is usually amenable to treatment if attended to almost immediately and resolves within a few days. We typically know exactly where, why, and how it hurts. For example, we feel pain at the location of an injury (cut, scrape, burn, fracture), surgical incision, toothache, or even an abdominal pain (appendicitis in the lower abdomen, pancreatitis and cholecystitis, in the upper abdomen).

Chronic pain

Pain lasting more than three months is classified as chronic. Sometimes it may be an acute pain becoming chronic but more often than not, the patient cannot clearly explain how, why, or when it started. The cause may be forgotten and the initiating injury or illness might have been too trivial to notice. Unlike acute pain, which most often originates from the periphery (skin or organs), chronic pain is assumed to be a disease of the nerves that carry the pain sensation. Chronic pain does not seem to have any protective action; on the contrary, the distress from it causes disability and disruption of various daily activities. Most of the pain management dilemmas and problems come from chronic pain and it is more difficult to treat because of the associated mental and emotional involvement.

How does pain become chronic?

Since pain serves the vital function of protecting the integrity of the body, nature has placed many failsafe mechanisms to ensure that pain is always felt, so that corrective and protective action can be taken. To understand how and why a protective and useful sensation like acute pain goes berserk to become an uncontrollable nuisance in chronic pain, it is necessary to recall that the pain pathway is a dynamic system that responds to increased traffic in various ways: it is subject to modulations all along the nervous systems, and finally in the brain as well. The CNS and PNS sensitizations can magnify not only the intensity and extent of pain but also the emotions associated with it. More importantly, sensitization has a self-sustaining capacity and is difficult to get rid of even after the original cause of the pain has been treated. Thus, chronic pain gets embedded in the pain pathway and the brain, and it becomes a disease in itself. The mind, being a part of the brain and the receptacle of the offshoots from the pain pathway, is as involved as the body in the experience of chronic pain.

Chronic pain differs significantly from acute pain as it entails more significant suffering. The distress of acute pain gets relieved the moment the physical pain is relieved and remains relieved unless there is an additional insult. Chronic pain, however, tends to lurk, linger, and recur for no reason at all except that it is the diseased nervous system revisiting itself, and is associated with a fear of recurrence and the associated anxiety and depression.

The gate control theory of pain

In 1965, Wall and Melzack[6] proposed the Gate Control Theory of Pain, which explains the protective nature of acute pain and the vagaries of chronic pain. They proposed that there are some specialized nerve cells in the spinal cord, which have the ability to either block or prioritize the incoming pain messages from the peripheral nerves. These neural gates monitor which messages should get through (or should not) to the brain—and at what speed and strength (Figure 7).

This gate is normally in a semi-closed condition, where mild pains only knock on it, and we continue to function normally. Moderate pain such as those from an abrasion or indigestion, are relayed more slowly or with less intensity. But a higher intensity, persistent pain can open the gate partially to ensure that it is felt, and protective action is taken. Severe pain (as in burns, which causes a barrage of impulses), is processed as an urgent warning, triggering the muscles, for example, to snatch the hand away from the stove (Figure 6).

Mechanisms of pain suppression

The body has many complementary mechanisms to suppress pain in highly-charged emergency or life-threatening situations.

- The neural gate helps the body in the fright-flight-fight response by suppressing even severe pains so that the animal or person can escape from danger.
- The pain of a gunshot may not be felt at the time because of immediate endorphin release but it is felt much later.

Endorphins are the natural "feel good" hormones that the body releases in large doses that help to relieve pain and can evince feelings of pleasure called euphoria. These are more potent than morphine although very similar in chemical structure. In fact, morphine is a very effective analgesic only because of its similarity to endorphin's chemical structure and it acts at many endorphin receptors in the body. Nature, the frugal resource manager, evolved a good chemical structure in morphine from plant-based opium, and then simply repeated it as a building block in later species, be it plant, animal, or human beings.

The gate control theory proposes that in chronic pain, the gate is continuously bombarded by pain impulses, which gradually nudge the gate to open more and more, till it is wide open. This "open gate" makes the pain pathway hypersensitive and is called spinal sensitization or "wind-up". A wide-open gate implies that even a mild pain will readily pass through to be perceived as being severe enough to breach the gate. Therefore, in chronic pain, the gate loses its discrimination, and pain perception loses its gradation, as all intensities of pain, mild to severe, are allowed to pass through. Consequently, all pains are felt as severe irrespective of their starting intensity, rather like a radio without a volume control, which just blares forth the moment it is switched on. In most chronic pains, the pain pathways in the PNS and CNS are persistently active. This sensitization amplifies the pain message out of proportion to the stimulus that causes the pain. For example, a patient with shingles (herpes) will jump even with a slight touch on the affected area. An interesting observation is that herpes is called *nagin* (snake) in India because of the way this painful stripe winds itself around the chest wall of the patient.

Often, the original disease or injury might have actually healed, but the spinal sensitization maintains the persistent activation in the pain pathways, to not only sustain the pain but also amplify it from stimuli that would not have bothered the person before the injury. This seemingly inexplicable aberrant behaviour of pain in neuropathy can be explained logically from the Ashirvad perspective of neuromyopathy which is discussed in the following chapters.

Further classification of pain

Both acute and chronic pain may be further classified as:

* Nociceptive and Neuropathic pain—depending on the cause.
* Somatic (body wall) and Visceral (organs) pain—depending on location

Nociceptive pain: In pain parlance, this indicates a pain caused by inflammation. The primary issue is in the tissues while the nerves show no structural damage. Nociceptive pain is usually well localized with a sharp, stabbing, throbbing, burning, stinging, tingling, nagging, dull or aching quality. It can be acute or chronic, mild or severe, or it can be somatic or visceral.

Somatic nociceptive pain: Arises from the skin, muscles, bones, joints, and is often aggravated by movement. Headaches, muscular pains, arthritis of joints due to ageing (osteoarthritis) and rheumatoid arthritis, all cause somatic nociceptive pains.

Visceral nociceptive pain: Occurs when the internal organs such as the gut, pancreas, lungs are inflamed or have a cancerous growth, or the involuntary heart muscle suffers compromised blood supply (ischaemia). In acute pancreatitis, the enzymes breach their natural location and start digesting tissues to cause chemical injury. Visceral pain is vague, ill-defined, dull aching and is often described as colicky.

Neuropathic pain: Defined as "pain caused by damage or disease affecting the somatosensory nervous system."[7] Somatosensory means sensory nerves that carry sensations from the somatic structures (skin, muscles, bones, and joints) to the CNS. It is the most common chronic pain occurring mainly due to nerve damage from ischaemia, infection, or injury, with aberrant pain messages being sent from nociceptors in PNS and/or CNS. Nerve damage could occur due to nerve entrapment between two taut muscles or between bone and muscle (Figure 5).

Radicular pain: Prolapse of the intervertebral disc causes neuropathic radicular pain by trapping the nerve root as it exits the spinal cord, against the vertebral bone (Figure 8). This pain combines nociceptive

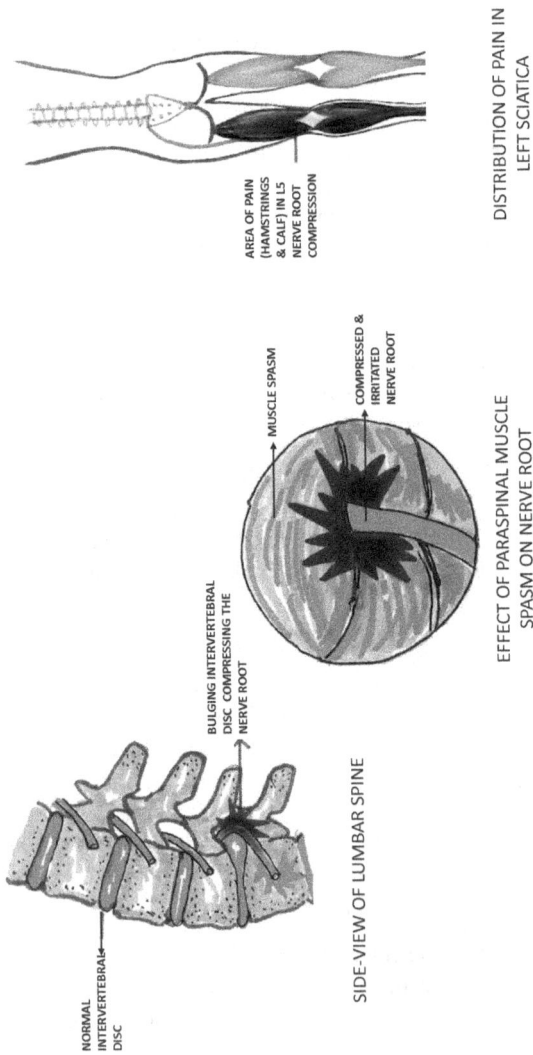

Figure 8. Sciatica caused by a prolapsed L4-5 intervertebral disc compressing the nerve and a second crush of the nerve between tight paraspinal muscles.

and neuropathic features. If the protruding disc damages the radicular nerve, then it is neuropathic pain. If the compression causes inflammation without nerve damage, it is nociceptive. It may be an acute disc prolapse or it may be chronic, where a previously healed disc prolapses again causing sciatica pain. Classical symptoms of radiculopathy (neuropathy of the radicular nerve) manifests with numbness, limb pain, weakness, and/or "pins and needles" sensation—among other symptoms. Further explanation and treatment are given in Chapter 3.

References

[1] Pirschel, C. 2018. Remembering Margo McCaffery's Contribution to Pain Management. ONS Voice.

[2] Raja, S.N., D.B. Carr, M. Cohen et al. 2020. The revised International Association for the Study of Pain definition of pain: concepts, challenges, and compromises. Pain 161(9): 1976–1982.

[3] Muller, J.P. 2011. Handbuch Der Physiologie Des Menschen: Für Vorlesungen. Reproduction. J. Hölscher, 1834. books.google.com.

[4] Ballantyne, J.C., S.M. Fishman and J.P. Rattmell et al. 2018. Bonica's Management of Pain. Wolters Kluwer Health, USA.

[5] Grunau, R.E., J.V. Miller and C.M. Chau et al. 2021. Long-term effects of pain in infants. pp. 38–46. *In*: Stevens, B.J., G. Hathway and W.T. Zemsky (eds.). Oxford Textbook of Pediatric Pain. https://academic.oup.com/book/35997.

[6] Melzack, R. and P.D. Wall. 1965. Pain mechanism: A new theory. Sci. 150(3699): 971–79.

[7] Treede, R.D., T.S. Jensen, J.N. Campbell et al. 2008. Neuropathic pain: redefinition and a grading system for clinical and research purposes. Neurology 70(18): 1630–1635.

Chapter 2

The Out-of-the-Box Approach

Most patients go to the family physician, physiotherapist, general physician, an orthopaedic surgeon, or a neurologist for pain treatment. Only when the pain remains unrelieved, do patients get referred to a pain specialist or they find one through personal contacts or the Internet. Over 70–80 per cent of our referrals come from previous patients.

Specific protocol

Step 1 is to record a detailed medical history, followed by a systematic physical examination of findings, and investigations. This protocol is identical to other pain clinics in India or abroad. The specific "treatment approach" diverges thereafter, because of our different and unique understanding of pain.

1. Detailed history

a) The intensity, quality, duration, constancy and location of pain are marked as a pictorial representation called the pain diagram (Figure 9). The emotional distress is specifically documented.

b) The baseline limitations in standing, walking, sitting, and other daily physical activities due to pain are documented for post-treatment comparison.

c) Previous pain history and interventions.

d) Any other pains elsewhere in the body.

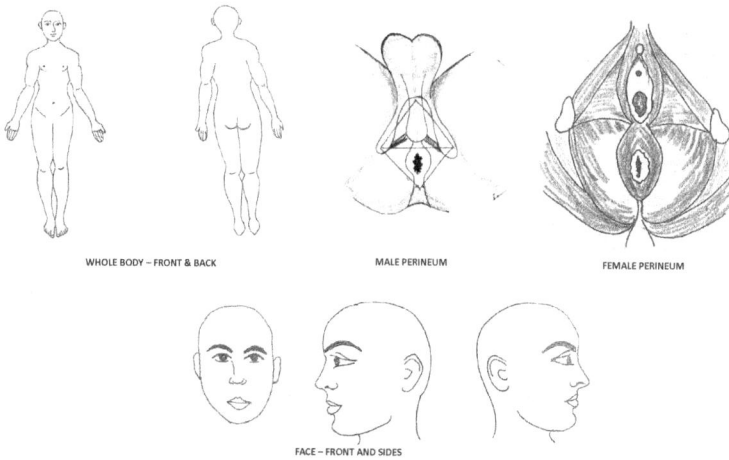

WHOLE BODY – FRONT & BACK   MALE PERINEUM   FEMALE PERINEUM

FACE – FRONT AND SIDES

Figure 9. Diagram of the body parts for the patients to mark their pain locations.

e) The general medical history to understand possible contribution from associated conditions (comorbidities), and drug interactions or possible side-effects.

f) A brief psychological profile of the patient includes an assessment of the general susceptibility to stress and whether there are any ongoing personal or professional tensions.

2. Examination

A thorough examination delineates the painful areas, tender areas, hypersensitive areas, and whether they correspond with the patient's description of the pain. Special attention is focused on documenting movement limitations with still photos and videos. For the patient's privacy facial photographs are avoided. For facial pains, the patient's consent is taken.

3. Investigations

A patient's history, examination, and investigations take time to document and provide sufficient information for a working diagnosis and to discuss the proposed treatment with the patient and family. Patients are routinely tested for deficiencies in vitamins B12 and D3 and C reactive protein, which indicates the presence of inflammatory processes that might explain the cause of pain. Additional investigations like X-rays, CT scans, and MRIs are done for locally-specific confirmation. Patients with severe pains may receive treatment the same day but usually, later appointments are given for treatment.

The out-of-the-box understanding of chronic pain

The treatment is primarily shaped by an unconventional understanding of pain itself rooted in the unique experiences with the initial lot of patients that we treated. These initial success outcomes have been repeatedly confirmed or validated in the subsequent years. Several scientific papers published on these concepts,[1-15] highlight the conceptual differences from the conventional world view.

There is still a significant amount of data, which awaits publication regarding the causes of common issues including locomotor and myofascial pain syndromes in areas such as the neck, shoulder, lower-back, sciatica and knee pain and conditions like headaches, migraines, post-surgical pain; and diverse uncommon pains encompassing neuropathy, neuralgias, central pain states, thoracoabdominal visceral pain, chronic pelvic pain, cancer-related pain, painful movement disorders like dystonia and even painless conditions like vertigo, persistent hiccups, and cerebral palsy.

The tried and tested old-fashioned approach: The unique evolution in our pain management in the first five years was rather like that of ancient physicians who had only the patient as the teacher to learn about diseases, medicines, and treatments. Even now, the focus is on closely observing the patients to get a sense of their psychophysical state and patiently listen to the important prologue of first-person inputs. Listening, observing, assessing, and figuring out the exact causes of the pain, workable treatments are formulated. The patients are made aware of the different Ashirvad understanding of pain and that the treatments are innovations, which have been effective in previous cases. It is emphasized that despite previous experiences of their efficacy, these treatments are not described in conventional pain books and therefore, prior consent for treatment is essential. After the treatment patients' feedbacks are documented, and the treatments are modified to suit the patients' needs once, twice, and yet again, as and when needed. This may sound presumptuous, but a fact that is reiterated daily is that assessment, diagnosis and treatment at Ashirvad results in an unequivocal positive response in 80–90 per cent of patients who have failed to improve with conventional pain treatments elsewhere. Sometimes it is a thorny, difficult road but fortunately, more often than not, it is a simpler road to complete recovery.

This successful understanding can be summed up briefly as below:

- All chronic pains develop a neuropathic component over time (nerve function disorder).

- All neuropathic pains involve the nerves that supply the muscles (the motor nerves) to develop a component of neuro-myo-pathy (muscle disorder + nerve disorder).

- Neuromyopathy causes major secondary muscle changes, which give rise to all confusing neuropathic pain symptoms.

- Therefore, unless the muscles, which are the main game players in *all* chronic pains are addressed as a priority, chronic pains are unlikely to be cured permanently and will keep recurring.

We first treat the involved nerves (both sensory and motor) and then specifically address the consequences of motor neuropathy by treating the muscles.

The realization that the muscle is the expressor of many pains has uncovered two extremely vital but poorly understood and unexplored aspects of chronic pain.

1. The disability associated with chronic pain is a primary manifestation of muscle disorder and not due to disuse as has been surmised. As the muscles are treated both the pain and disability get reversed simultaneously. As a corollary, many painless muscle disorders also respond.

2. *The mind-muscle connection*: Nature seems to have placed a veritable freeway between the mind and muscle probably because the muscle is the prime mover for the execution of the lifesaving fright-flight-fight response. The muscles are the first responders in this essential survival reflex and are equipped with adequate nerve and blood supply, which not only propels the muscle into instant action but also dilates the blood vessels to provide adequate nutritional and oxygen resources to perform quick action. Because the mind and muscle are the two integral components of this reflex, every emotion has some reflection on the muscle. Anger, fear, anxiety, resentment, or even continuous work tensions singularly or collectively, all increase muscle tension, particularly around the areas of pre-existing pain. When the mind is stressed, the muscles around the pain area are held tight, exacerbating the pain intensity or widening the pain distribution. The converse is also true with

patients who are calm, their pain levels decrease. The muscles are the intermediate media through which the mind influences pain, worsening it by the increased muscle spasms or decreasing the pain by relaxing the painful muscles as during distraction, meditation, mindfulness, or autosuggestion. What happens in the muscle is continuously communicated to the CNS at both the conscious (cognition) and unconscious (proprioception) levels. Proprioception or kinaesthesia is the brain's unconscious/conscious ability to sense the body's posture and disposition of the body parts as well as their movement, action, and location. It is most essential for maintaining posture and balance. For example, while we are eating, the hand goes from the plate to the mouth automatically; yet we are unaware of the hand holding the spoon and where exactly it is positioned in its transit from the plate to the mouth unless we consciously make it a point to become aware. Yoga uses this technique of diverting awareness from the mind's non-essential (and often unreal and detrimental) chatter to conscious awareness of bodily activities of daily life. Yoga *asana*s, divert the mind's focus to the posture and breathing or breathing alone in respiratory or meditative practices, which direct (or divert in case of pain) the mind inwards, away from the painful area, thereby helping in reducing pain.

Our out-of-the-box treatment integrates the two-fold targets of addressing pain/disability and the muscle/mind axis, to empower patients by introducing them to the power of their mind in influencing or managing pain be it with counselling, mindfulness, yoga, or a psychological referral.

Understanding neuropathic pain

The successful reversal of many terrible pain conditions over the past 20 years was possible because we acknowledged that all neuropathic pains are neuromyopathic.

Nerves are traditionally divided into three categories:

- Purely motor or efferent nerves travel *away from* the spinal cord to supply muscles, for example, facial nerve.
- Purely sensory or afferent nerves travel *towards* the spinal cord from all over the body. For example, the medial cutaneous nerve of the arm.

- Mixed nerves combine the sensory and motor nerves with impulses travelling both *towards* and *away from* the spinal cord. These comprise most nerves in the body.

The international definition of neuropathic pain as, "Pain caused by damage or disease affecting the somatosensory nervous system,"[16] excludes the whole gamut of the motor nervous system from neuropathy. However, it is evident that the motor nerves are as affected by neuropathy as the somatosensory nervous system.

The muscle is a highly sensitive organ with a multitude of free nerve endings capable of picking up and transmitting many sensations, mainly temperature and pain. Anyone who has had a muscle cramp or a crick in the neck knows the severe pain that a muscle can generate. Thus, a 'pure' motor nerve must contain nerves with bidirectional traffic; the efferent nerves *from* the spinal cord, which make the muscle contract and the afferent musculo-sensory and proprioceptive nerves that carry muscle pain and other sensations *to* the spinal cord (Figure 10).

Motor nerves are as vulnerable to neuropathy as sensory nerves. The sensory nerves act more like passive conduits in pain transmission while the motor nerves or the motor fibres in a mixed nerve affected by neuropathy are the root cause for the ubiquitous finding of myofascial

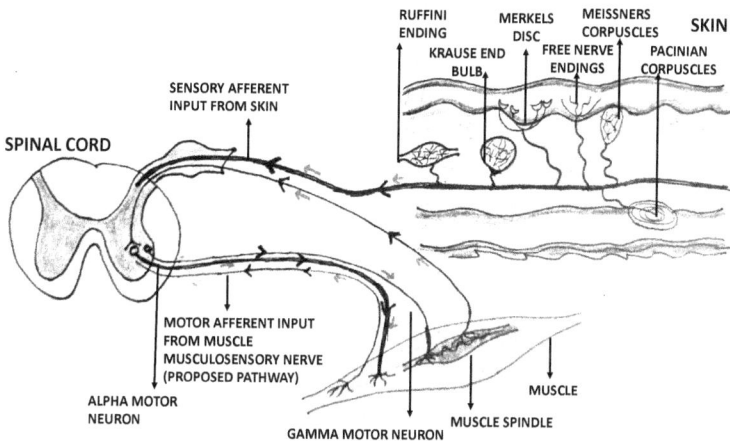

Figure 10. Top right: Unidirectional afferent pain transmission from the skin receptors to spinal cord. Bottom right: Bidirectional transmission. Efferent fibres from the spinal cord cause muscle contraction while the afferent musculo-sensory fibres go towards the spinal cord.

pain syndrome (MPS) in most chronic pain conditions. This vital insight is missing in the current understanding of pain. The exclusion of a major part of the nervous system, the motor nerves, in the definition of neuropathy has influenced the pain management think tanks across the world to turn a blind eye to the motor nerves and muscles. This has led to a situation where most current interventions in pain management are confined to the somatosensory nervous system. In practice, MPS is extremely common and reportedly accounts for more than 85 per cent of chronic pain.[17–19] but has been explained as an associated finding (comorbidity) in chronic pains.[20] No wonder that current treatments that focus exclusively on the somatosensory nervous system have failed to yield good outcomes.

The Ashirvad understanding of neuropathy as neuromyopathy represents a paradigm shift in this basic concept of pain and has led to the evolution of the out-of-the-box innovation called ultrasound guided dry needling (USGDN) (Figure 11). Its predecessors, intramuscular stimulation (IMS)[21] and dry needling, (DN)[22] were quasi-effective with unsustained efficacy. How this was honed and developed into a scientific and highly effective treatment with the introduction of the ultrasound visualization is explained in detail in Chapter 3.

Mechanism of muscle involvement in neuropathy

The neuromuscular junction (NMJ) is the site where the terminal branches of motor nerves spread out to contact muscle fibre groups. The nerve and the muscle fibres that it innervates form a motor unit (Figure 12). Groups of motor units work together to coordinate the contractions of a single muscle.

Excessive firing at the NMJ by a neuropathic motor nerve, causes sustained erratic contractions of several motor units depending on the level of nerve irritability. The two sliding components of the muscle fibre called actin and myosin do not return to their original position away from one another and get fixed in the contracted position, to form muscle knots called myofascial trigger points (MTrPs) in muscle fibres (Figure 13). MTrPs may be initially non-painful (latent MTrPs) but inflammatory mediators collect around a MTrP to make it spontaneously painful (active MTrPs)[24–29] and make muscle movements painful (Figures 14, 15). The plentiful polymodal free nerve endings, which are spread-out all-over the muscles, are capable of carrying the pain sensation from the MTrPs to the spinal cord and brain. Inflammatory mediators also

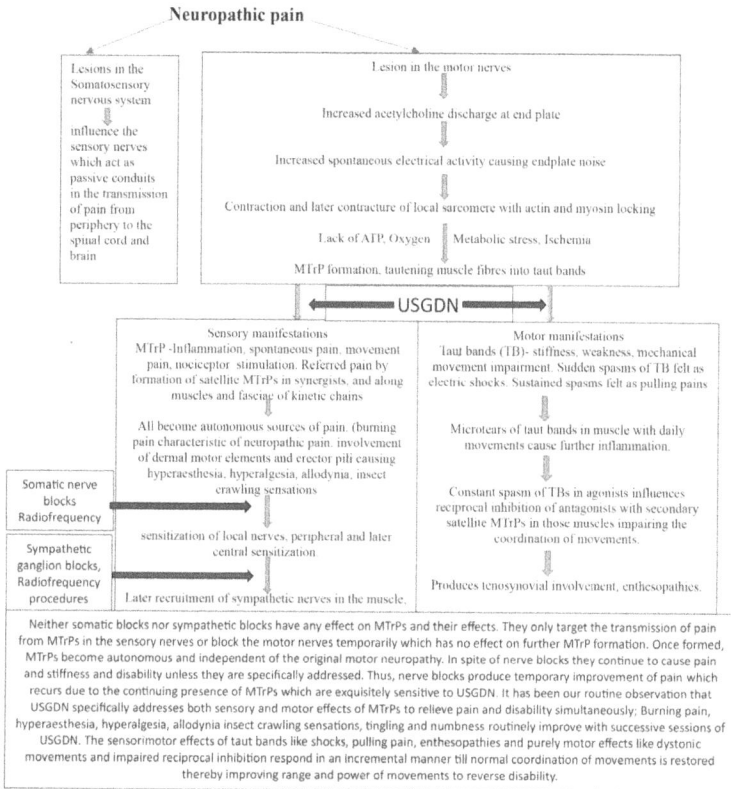

Figure 11. A diagrammatic representation of a working hypothesis to explain neuromyopathy; sequence of events leading to MTrP generation, production of inflammatory mediators, consequences of MTrP and taut bands. The relevance of neural blocks and USGDN in this sequence of events and the significance of USGDN in neuropathic pains is shown. Figure taken from Reference 1 with permission.

enhance the pain impulse conduction to produce peripheral sensitization and subsequent central sensitization.[28, 29]

Once formed, the MTrPs become independent of the nerve irritation that generated them in the first place, and autonomously continue to cause pain even after motor neuropathy has resolved and motor nerve firing at the NMJ has ceased. Persistence of MTrPs and their sequelae seems to be the rule in every type of neuromyopathy where the nerve irritation initiates the formation of MTrPs, which then continue to produce persistent pain despite the neuropathy healing as it happens in herpes and after "successful surgery" on the back, knee, abdomen, or

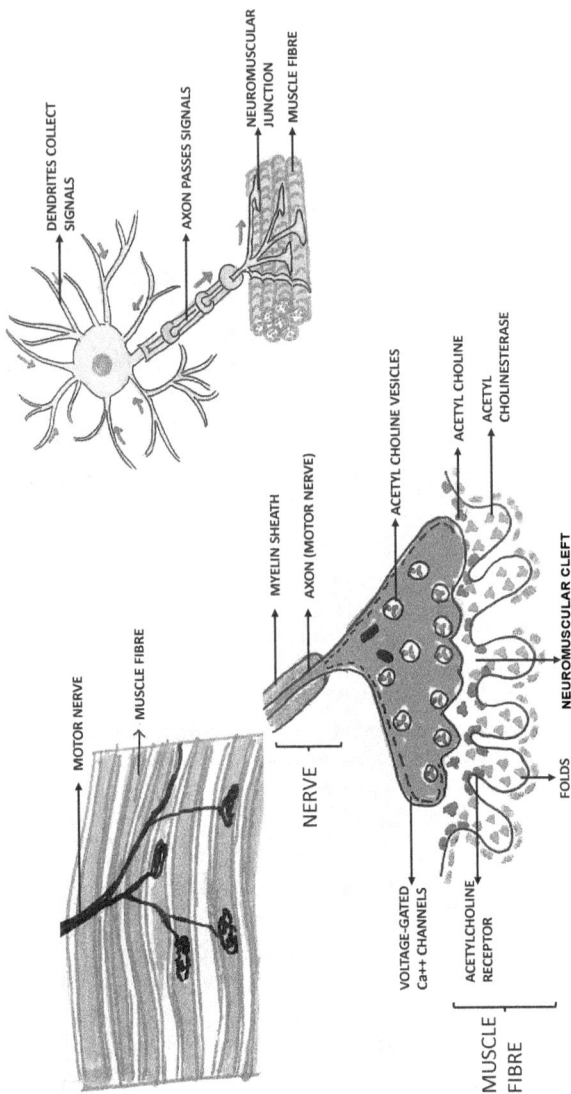

Figure 12. Top left: Motor neuron innervating muscle fibres (motor unit). Right: Motor nerve innervating many motor units.Bottom: Neuron meets the muscle at the neuromuscular junction.

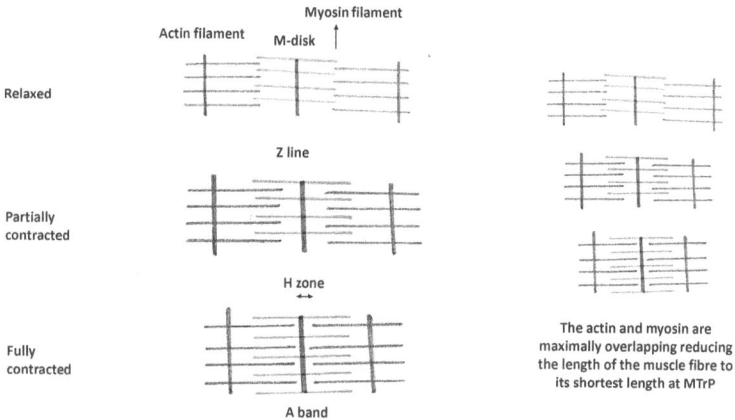

Figure 13. Actin and myosin overlap shortens the muscle during contraction. A persistent and unrelieved contracture/spasm generates myofascial trigger points (MTrPs).

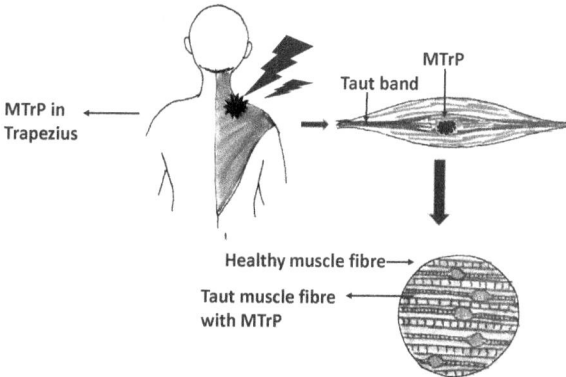

Figure 14. MTrPs causing pain, muscle shortening, and taut bands.

a craniotomy, and even after pain management procedures like nerve blocks, RF, and spinal card stimulators.

The presence of multiple MTrPs tautens the muscle fibres and over time, shortens them (Figures 14, 15). These taut bands understandably, are responsible for the motor features; the recruitment of agonist/antagonist muscle combinations get impaired to impede smooth execution of movements. Taut bands contract preferentially before the surrounding normal muscle fibres as determined by a physiological law called the Starling's Law[5, 23] to produce stiffness coupled with weakness, a hallmark complaint of all chronic pains.

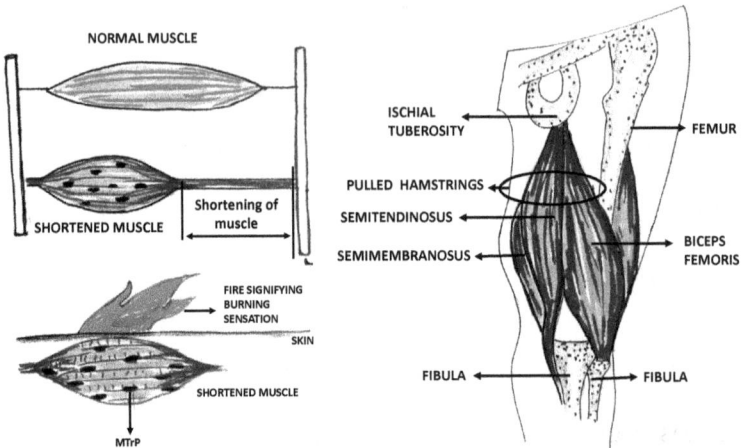

Figure 15. Top left: Normal muscle compared with one shortened by MTrPs and taut bands. Right: Taut bands cause a pulled, painful, hamstring. Bottom left: MTrPs stimulate temperature receptors to refer burning pain to the overlying skin.

MTrPs can also express pain at a distant point in the hand or foot, called pain referral. This occurs because fascia covering individual muscles extends down the limb connecting the muscles in the arm, forearm, and hand to form a continuous action chain, which travels across the limb. Since no muscle works in isolation, for every action, groups of muscles have to work together. This functional connection between muscles, the kinetic chain, leads to a domino effect where the impedance of one muscle action by taut bands will impede the contractions and function of all the muscles in the kinetic chain down the limb, which carry out the same action or oppose it. The ensuing embarrassment produces a painful line of satellite MTrPs in the coworking muscle groups down the limb culminating in variegated MPSs, which are ubiquitous in most chronic pain states with motor neuropathy. For instance, if the bicep has taut bands impeding its action, the muscles that bend the elbow, wrist, and fingers and lift the shoulders have to work harder or work awkwardly to perform the act of conveying food from the plate to the mouth. Similarly, MTrPs in the buttock muscles generate painful MTrPs in the muscles along the thigh, leg, and foot.

But by far the most confusing feature of painful taut bands are the myriad confounding *sensory* features of chronic pain in neuropathic conditions,[30] like burning, shocks, tenderness, pain referral down the limb and allodynia (where a light touch is felt as pain). Ultrasound guided dry needling (USGDN), which specifically resolves MTrPs, consistently and astoundingly reverses the sensorimotor symptoms of many so-called incurable conditions, even those, which are said to exclusively involve the sensory nerves, like herpes zoster, trigeminal neuralgia, CRPS types 1 and 2, post-stroke pains, and brachial plexus injuries. This understanding has revolutionized the approach to these conditions, leading to the development of many innovative therapies (discussed in the next chapter) which avoid highly invasive and expensive interventions or opioid prescriptions for providing pain relief.

Classic sensory features of neuropathy and USGDN

The following is a brief explanation of the genesis of the crippling, distressing symptoms in neuropathic pain and how they respond, routinely and invariably, to USGDN repeatedly confirming the concept of neuromyopathy.

Pulling pain: Painful taut bands cause an actual pull during normal movements (Figure 15). For example, hamstring pain in radiculopathy from disc prolapse, pulls at its origin in the ischial tuberosity in buttocks, along the back of the thigh, and behind the knee at its insertion. Pains recur after an epidural steroid injection when the patient attempts to increase standing and walking. But 10–12 USGDN sessions progressively decrease and eliminate these pulling pains, even after walking for an hour. The clockwork-like precision of the response allows the patient to increase physical activities with the confidence that USGDN will relieve all pain recurrences and overcome the disability to revert to the prior lifestyle.

Burning: Since our body temperature is maintained by the heat from muscular activity, nature has provided enough temperature receptors in the muscles to provide feedback to the brain's temperature-control centre. We believe that these polymodal receptors, which are sensitive to both pain and temperature, are stimulated by the inflammatory pain from an active MTrP and the abnormally constant and intense contraction of multiple taut bands. This generates a deep muscular pain and a burning sensation in the overlying skin (Figure 15). This condition of the pain and burning sensation is routinely treated with USGDN.

Skin hypersensitivity: Muscle elements are present in the dermis of the skin to impart the suppleness of youth and wrinkles later in life. Erector pili are skin muscles specifically organized around a hair follicle to raise the hair during cold or fear, causing 'goosebumps' (Figure 16). We believe that intense dermal muscle spasm causes a local inflammation under the skin making it extremely tender and hypersensitive, rendering a normal and certainly painless touch to be perceived as painful (allodynia) and a mild pain is felt as severe pain (hyperalgesia). In herpes, pain from intense intercostal muscle spasms is referred to the skin muscles to cause allodynia and hyperalgesia making even the touch of clothes or the mild fan breeze intolerable. USGDN routinely reverses these symptoms by targeting the dermal muscles enroute to the deeper intercostal muscles.

Insect crawling: Irregular flickers of the dermal muscle fibres trigger the 'creepy' sensation of an insect crawling under the skin (Figure 16). Skin hypersensitivity and the insect crawling sensation are the first symptoms that respond to USGDN.

Numbness: Nerves travel in intermuscular compartments (Figure 17) and can get compressed/entrapped by muscle spasms to cause severe pain and numbness typical of neuropathy. Terminal skin branches travelling through taut bands to the skin get compressed to cause numbness with a normal touch sensation. Usually there may be no demonstrable nerve damage, but prolonged entrapment, injury, or cancerous invasion can devitalize a nerve. This classic neuropathic paradoxical manifestation of pain in an area of numbness is routinely reversed by USGDN, although the pain responds before the numbness. Recovery may be partial or absent in actual nerve damage.

Electric shock-like sensations: These are apparently caused by the sudden severe contraction of few taut bands within the muscle, like the sudden yanking of a strand of hair. Shocks routinely respond to USGDN.

To summarize, muscles with MTrPs are not just pain generators but also expressors and sustainers of nerve pain making them the final common tool for the expression of pain in practically all the chronic pains. Consistent success in reversing various types of difficult and hitherto untreatable symptoms and conditions has confirmed that nature has chosen to combine the dual tools of survival, pain and muscles, which execute the fright, flight, or fight reflex to safeguard the physical body.

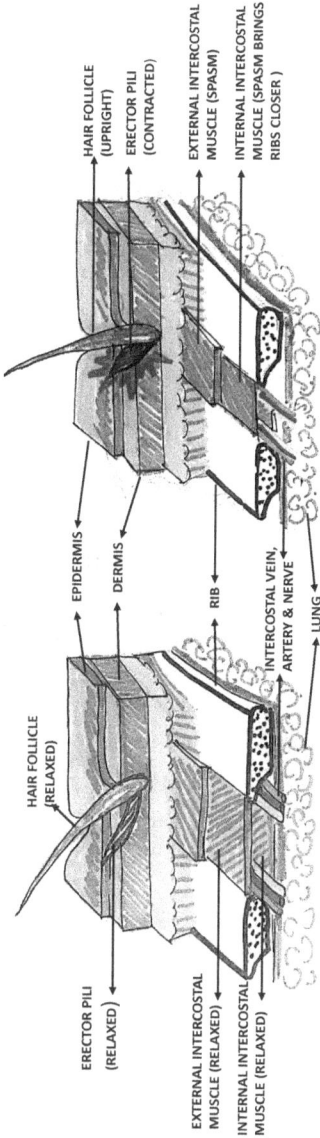

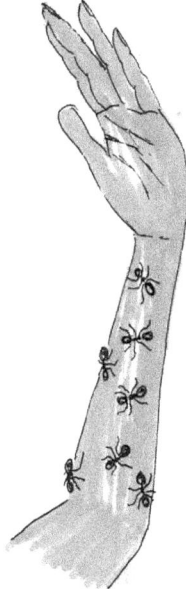

Figure 16. Top left: Skin muscle at the hair root, erector pili, relaxed. Right: Contracts to raise the hair (goose bumps). Intense spasm of skin muscles and the more deeply located intercostal muscles cause the skin hypersensitivity and burning in herpes. Bottom: Intermittent irregular contractions of the tiny skin muscle fibres causing an insect-crawling sensation in the skin.

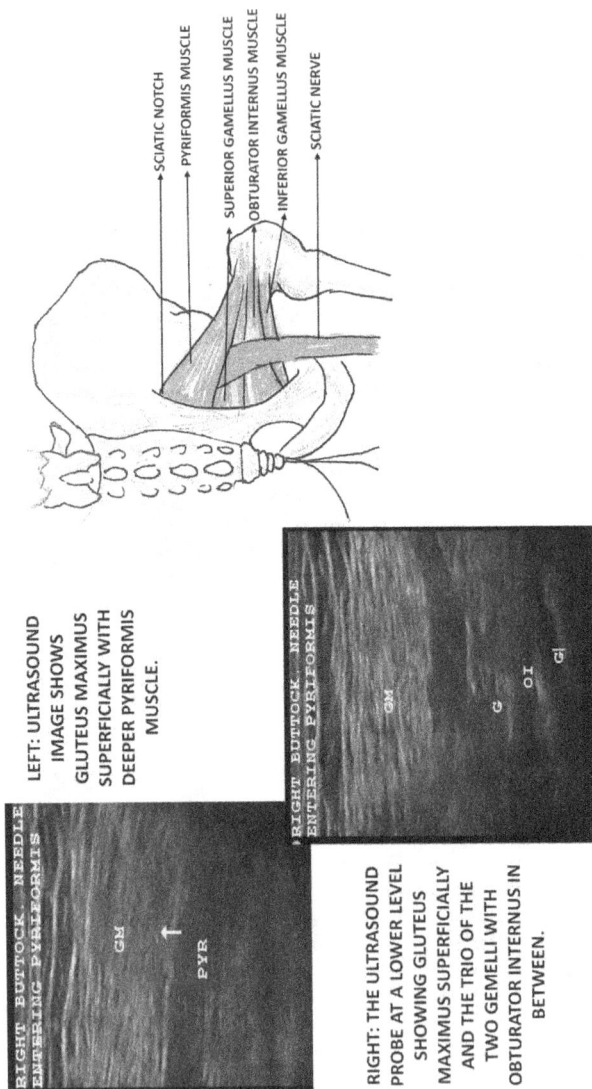

Figure 17. Top left: Needle (white arrow) in the gluteus maximus (GM) and piriformis (PYR) muscle. Right: The piriformis and the superior gemellus muscle entrap the sciatic nerve in sciatica. Bottom: The lower gluteus maximus (GM) overlies the superior and inferior gemelli muscles (G) with the obturator internus (OI) in between.

An exquisitely frugal manager, nature uses muscles as the universal building blocks in variegated forms to generate, convey, and sustain a mind-boggling array of pains.

References

[1] Vas, L.C. 2022. Ultrasound guided dry needling: Relevance in chronic pain. J. Postgrad. Med. Jan 1; 68(1): 1.

[2] Vas, L. 2019. Effectiveness of ultrasound guided dry needling in chronic pain. Pain News 17(4): 202–212.

[3] Vas, L. and R. Pai. 2019. Ultrasound guided dry needling as a treatment for postmastectomy pain syndrome—A case series of twenty patients. Indian J. Palliat Care 25(1): 93–102.

[4] Vas, L., S. Phanse and R. Pai. 2016. A new perspective of neuromyopathy to explain intractable pancreatic cancer pains; dry needling as an effective adjunct to neurolytic blocks. Indian J. Palliat Care 22(1): 85–93.

[5] Vas, L., R. Pai, N. Khandagale et al. 2015. Myofascial trigger points as a cause of abnormal co-contraction in writer's cramp. Pain Med. 16(10): 2041–2045.

[6] Vas, L., N. Khandagale and R. Pai et al. 2014. Successful management of chronic postsurgical pain following total knee replacement. Pain Med. 15(10): 1781–1785.

[7] Vas, L., N. Khandagale, R. Pai et al. 2014. Pulsed radiofrequency of the composite nerve supply to the knee joint as a new technique for relieving osteoarthritic pain: A preliminary report. Pain Physician 17: 493–506.

[8] Vas, L., M. Patnaik, V. Walker et al. 2014. Treatment of a patient with interstitial cystitis/painful bladder syndrome as a neuropathic pain condition with a combination of caudal epidural analgesia followed by Botox injection of perineal muscles. Indian Journal of Urology 30.3: 350.

[9] Vas, L., S. Phanse, K.S. Pawar et al. 2023. Ultrasound guided dry needling of masticatory muscles in trigeminal neuralgia—A case series of 35 patients. J. Postgrad. Med. 69: 11–20.

[10] Vas, L., R. Pai, K.S. Pawar et al. 2016. "Piriformis Syndrome": Is it only Piriformis? Pain Med. 17(9): 1775–1779.

[11] Vas, L. 2006. How to set up a pain clinic and practice as a pain management specialist. A review article. Indian J. Anaesth 50(5): 408–415.

[12] Sharma, M., S. Gupta and L. Vas et al. 2022. Mesothelioma and chest wall pain. pp. 63–74. *In*: Sharma, M., K.H. Simpson, M.I. Bennett et al. (eds.). Practical Management of Complex Cancer Pain. 2nd ed. Oxford University Press, London.

[13] Vas, L. 2022. Unilateral upper limb plexopathy pain caused by cancer. pp. 75–86. *In*: Sharma, M., K.H. Simpson, M.I. Bennett et al. (eds.). Practical Management of Complex Cancer Pain. 2nd ed. Oxford University Press, London.

[14] Sharma, M. and L. Vas. 2022. Interventions for head and neck cancer related pain. pp. 261–274. *In*: Sharma, M., K.H. Simpson, M.I. Bennett et al. (eds.). Practical Management of Complex Cancer Pain. 2nd ed. Oxford University Press, London.

[15] Vas, L., M. Sharma and S. Gupta et al. 2022. Peripheral nerve blocks including neurolytic blocks. pp. 285–292. *In*: Sharma, M., K.H. Simpson, M.I. Bennett et al. (eds.). Practical Management of Complex Cancer Pain. 2nd ed. Oxford University Press, London.

[16] Treede, R.D., T.S. Jensen, J.N. Campbell et al. 2008. Neuropathic pain: Redefinition and a grading system for clinical and research purposes. Neurology 70: 1630–1635.

[17] Gunn, C.C. 2001. Neuropathic myofascial pain syndromes. pp. 522–529. *In*: Bonica's Management of Pain. Lippincott Williams & Wilkins, Philadelphia, USA.

[18] Gattie, E., J.A. Cleland and S. Snodgrass et al. 2017. The effectiveness of trigger point dry needling for musculoskeletal conditions by physical therapists: A systematic review and meta-analysis. J. Orthop Sports Phys. Ther. 47: 133–149.

[19] Vulfsons, S. and A. Minerbi. 2020. The case for comorbid myofascial pain—A qualitative review. Int. J. Environ. Res. Public Health 17: 5188.

[20] Fishbain, D.A., M. Goldberg, B.R. Meagher et al. 1986. Male and female chronic pain patients categorized by DSM-III psychiatric diagnostic criteria. Pain 26: 181–197.

[21] Skootsky, S.A., B. Jaeger and R.K. Oye et al. 1989. Prevalence of myofascial pain in general internal medicine practice. West J. Med. 151: 157–160.

[22] Gerwin, R.D. 2001. Classification, epidemiology, and natural history of myofascial pain syndrome. Curr. Pain Headache Rep. 5: 412–420.

[23] Travell, J.G. and D.G. Simons. 1983. Myofascial Pain and Dysfunction: The Trigger Point Manual. Lippincott Williams & Wilkins, Philadelphia, USA.

[24] Arendt-Nielsen, L. and M. Castaldo. 2015. MTPs are a peripheral source of nociception. Pain Med. 16: 625–627.

[25] Dommerholt, J. and P. Huijbregts (eds.). 2010. Myofascial Trigger Points: Pathophysiology and Evidence-informed Diagnosis and Management. Jones & Bartlett Learning, Burlington, USA.

[26] Jin, F., Y. Guo, Z. Wang et al. 2020. The pathophysiological nature of sarcomeres in trigger points in patients with myofascial pain syndrome: A preliminary study. Eur. J. Pai. 24: 1968–1978.

[27] Chen, Q., H-j. Wang, R.E. Gay et al. 2016. Quantification of myofascial taut bands. Arch Phys. Med. Rehabil. 97: 67–73.

[28] Shah, J.P., N. Thaker, J. Heimur et al. 2015. Myofascial trigger points then and now: A historical and scientific perspective. PM&R 7: 746–761.

[29] Sikdar, S., J.P. Shah, T. Gebreab et al. 2009. Novel applications of ultrasound technology to visualize and characterize myofascial trigger points and surrounding soft tissue. Arch Phys. Med. Rehabil. 90: 1829–1838.

[30] Mense, S. 2003. The pathogenesis of muscle pain. Curr. Pain Headache Rep. 7: 419–425.

Chapter 3

Treatment Protocols

The uniqueness of the Ashirvad treatment protocol is that disability is given as much importance as pain relief. As soon as pain is relieved (usually within a week or two), the focus shifts to reducing/relieving the disability, so that patients can gradually return to a normal active lifestyle. The sole purpose of the treatment is to bring the patients to the active lifestyle that they had prior to the onset of pain.

Conservative treatments

Medications

Oral medication is the most basic treatment, easy for the patient to take and for doctors to prescribe. Common pain medication falls into three categories:[1]

1. *Painkillers or basic analgesics*: They have an anti-inflammatory effect at the nociceptors and along the pain pathway.

2. *Other analgesic medications*: They act on the receptors for neurochemicals, opioids, and cannabinoids, in the PNS and CNS. They may either be non-opioid or mild/powerful opioid medications.

3. *Neuromodulators*: They influence the electrochemical activity in the pain pathway and its interconnections—the rationale for managing pain with these medications:

   • *The electrical impulses*: Electrical impulses carrying the pain messages are mediated by fluctuations of calcium, sodium, and potassium ions across the nerve cell membranes. The wonder drugs of anaesthesia, the local anaesthetics, block the sodium channels to cause sensorimotor suppression. Anticonvulsant drugs like pregabalin and gabapentin block the alpha 2 delta calcium channels to inhibit the onward impulse progression in the pain pathway.

• Medications may also facilitate or inhibit the impulses coming from the higher brain centres to the pain pathway by conserving, augmenting, or depleting the level of CNS neurotransmitters to produce complex effects on pain. For example, antidepressants like venlafaxine, duloxetine and the synthetic opioid tramadol influence major neurotransmitters like noradrenaline, serotonin, and dopamine.

4. *Opioids*: These act on opioid receptors, which Nature places at strategic points of the pain pathway to respond to the enkephalins and endorphins that our bodies produce. Their efficacy relies majorly on a sense of detachment from the unpleasantness of pain called 'affect', and either a sense of euphoria (well-being or happiness), or dysphoria (discomfort or distress), depending on which opioid receptor they act on.

5. *Miscellaneous medications*: The prominent medications are muscle relaxants, antidepressants, prescribed for their effect at the pain pathway (depression requires a much higher dose), anxiolytics, sedatives, local anaesthetics, and others: anaesthetic medications like N methyl D aspartate blockers, dexmedetomidine and ketamine, alfa2 receptor blockers like clonidine with major effects on pain transmission.

The treatment starts with a medication combination (analgesics, both non-opioid and opioid as indicated+neuromodulators±muscle relaxants± any other medications as indicated). Pain reduction by 10–30 per cent is considered a positive response. Most patients are initially happy with this respite but naturally, with time, want more relief. Besides, medications have side-effects like acidity, nausea, vomiting, constipation, and drowsiness. Opioids and cannabinoids also have the risk of dependence and addiction.

Physical therapy (PT)

Physiotherapy has been the consistent mainstay of pain management along with medication.[2] Most pains involve the muscles and hence respond to physiotherapy to some extent. If the patients improve enough to resume a normal lifestyle, then PT is all they need. But unfortunately, in many chronic pain conditions, improvement peters out after the initial 20–30 per cent relief. For such patients, referral to a pain specialist is most beneficial. The armamentarium of treatments available at our disposal in addition to PT can custom-design treatments for all pains, as discussed in this chapter.

Interventional treatment

These are routinely performed in most pain clinics[3,4] and can be classified as:

* Basic interventions.
* Advanced and invasive interventions, which may have hardware to be implanted in the body, and hence are more expensive.[5–7]

USGDN is a unique intervention that is an exclusive part of the Ashirvad treatment, which addresses the myofascial contribution to pain and disability. Basic and/or advanced interventions to address the neural component of pain are followed by USGDN to address the invariable culprit in all chronic pains, the ubiquitous muscle involvement. Many patients with predominant MPS improve with only USGDN along with correction of vitamin deficiencies, medication, and PT. This approach, therefore, provides the flexibility of offering USGDN as a stand-alone treatment or as an additional treatment that prolongs the effects of basic and advanced neural interventions for complete and long-lasting relief from pain and disability.

Basic neural interventions

Nerve blocks: injections that target a nerve in PNS or CNS.

a) *Single peripheral nerve* (PNS): These are useful when pain is confined to the distribution of one nerve. For example, ulnar or sciatic nerve block (Figure 18).

b) *Plexus nerves* (PNS): Most pains occur in parts of the body like the limbs or face. A brachial plexus block covers all the upper limb nerves (Figure 18).

In addition to the sensory and motor nerves that are under voluntary control there are innumerable sympathetic/parasympathetic nerves of the autonomic or involuntary nervous system, which are not under voluntary

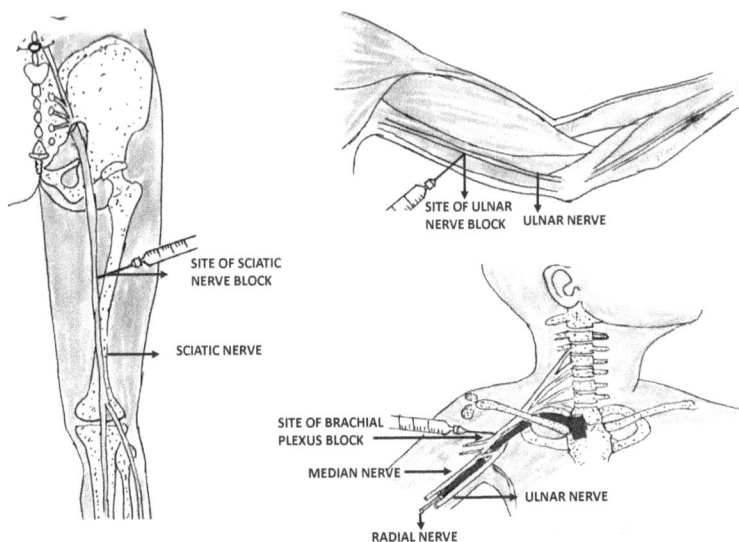

Figure 18. Sciatic and ulnar nerve blocks and brachial plexus block.

control. These converge and communicate with each other in relay stations called the sympathetic/parasympathetic ganglia:

- Stellate ganglion for the sympathetic nerves of the head, face, neck, and upper limbs.
- Celiac ganglion for abdominal sensations.
- Hypogastric ganglia for pelvic pains.
- Lumbar sympathetic ganglion for the lower limbs.

By injecting a local anaesthetic and steroid near the sympathetic ganglia it is possible to suppress the sympathetically mediated pain that it relays. X-ray guidance shows the drug spread with radio-opaque dye while ultrasonography visualization minimizes the risks by accurately pinpointing the exact position of the needle tip and the medicine spreading (Figure 19).

c) *The spinal cord* (CNS): Epidural injections or spinal nerve root block are the most commonly performed procedures for back and neck pains, radiating down the limb. Back pain is among the most common pain conditions presented to pain clinics. It may be due to intervertebral disc issues, facet joint issues, age-related

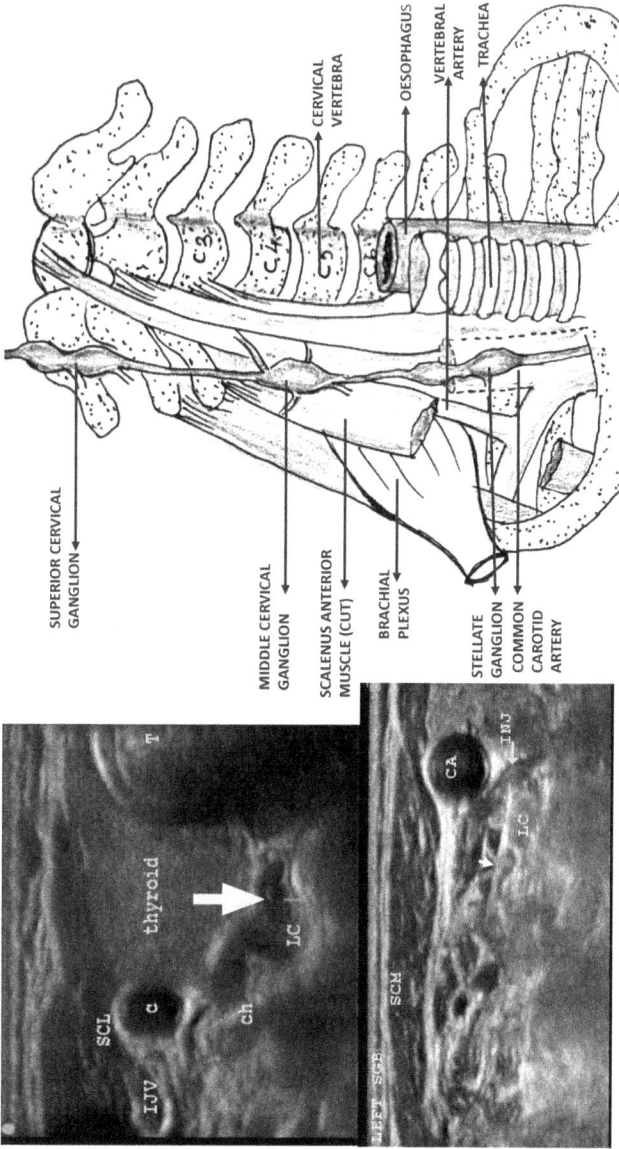

Figure 19. Top left: Stellate ganglion (white arrow) on the Longus Colli (LC) muscle. Bottom left: The white arrow shows the needle with the pool of the local anaesthetic (INJ) at the stellate ganglion. Right: diagrammatic representation of sympathetic ganglia in the neck and the brachial plexus. SCL – sternocleidomastoid muscle; IJV – internal jugular vein; C, CA – carotid; ch – Chassaignac's tubercle; T – trachea.

degenerative changes in the spine, and so on. Disc or facet pathology compromises the radicular nerve, which emerges from the spinal cord and gives off numerous branches in the back and down the limb to innervate specific muscles. An injection around the spinal cord at the emergence of the radicular nerve (transforaminal epidural block) or around the radicular nerve (nerve root block) is required to relieve the back pain and the radicular pain extending down the limb (Figures 8, 20).

Regenerative therapies: utilize platelet rich plasma and other stem cells which are extracted from the patient's own blood or body tissues to be injected with pinpoint accuracy under ultrasound visualization into painful areas to initiate regeneration of tissues in joints, muscles and ligaments.

Advanced interventions

A) Radiofrequency (RF) procedures (continuous RF, pulsed RF, and cooled RF).[5]

B) Continuous nerve block (CNB) techniques.

C) Intrathecal pump (ITP).[6]

D) Spinal cord stimulators (SCS) and dorsal root ganglion stimulation (DRG Stim).[7]

A) *Radiofrequency (RF) procedures*

This is an extremely efficacious and useful intervention for addressing the neural component of pain. It requires a radiofrequency generator, a grounding pad, an electrode placed in an insulated cannula with an uninsulated tip to convey the RF current to the nerve (Figure 21). The RF current causes agitation and oscillation of tissue molecules around the nerve, which generates heat. The thermocouple at the electrode tip senses this and reflects it on the RF generator screen for controlling the temperature at the desired level.

Three types of RF are used in pain medicine:

a) *Continuous/conventional/thermal   radiofrequency* (commonly referred to as thermal RF) delivers a continuous RF energy leading to a steady temperature increase up to 80–90°C to produce a 4 mm elliptical burn of the nerve segment exposed to the uninsulated RF needle tip (Figure 22). The burnt nerve segment cannot conduct

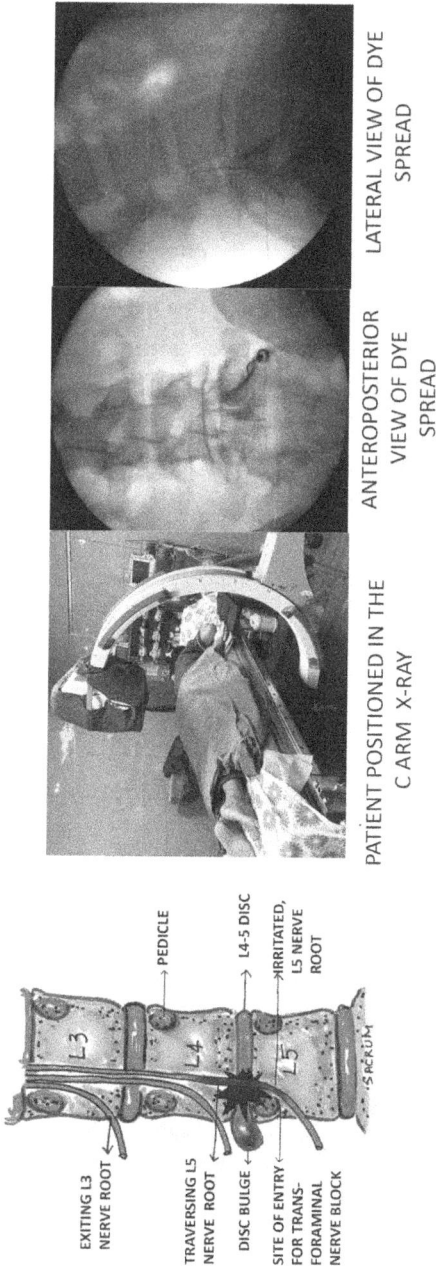

Figure 20. Left: Lumbar L3, L4, L5 nerve roots exit beneath the respective vertebral pedicles. The exiting L5 nerve root compressed by L4-L5 disc (black). Middle: Patient positioned under the C-Arm X-ray. Right: Black radio-opaque dye around L5 nerve root seen on back and the side view.

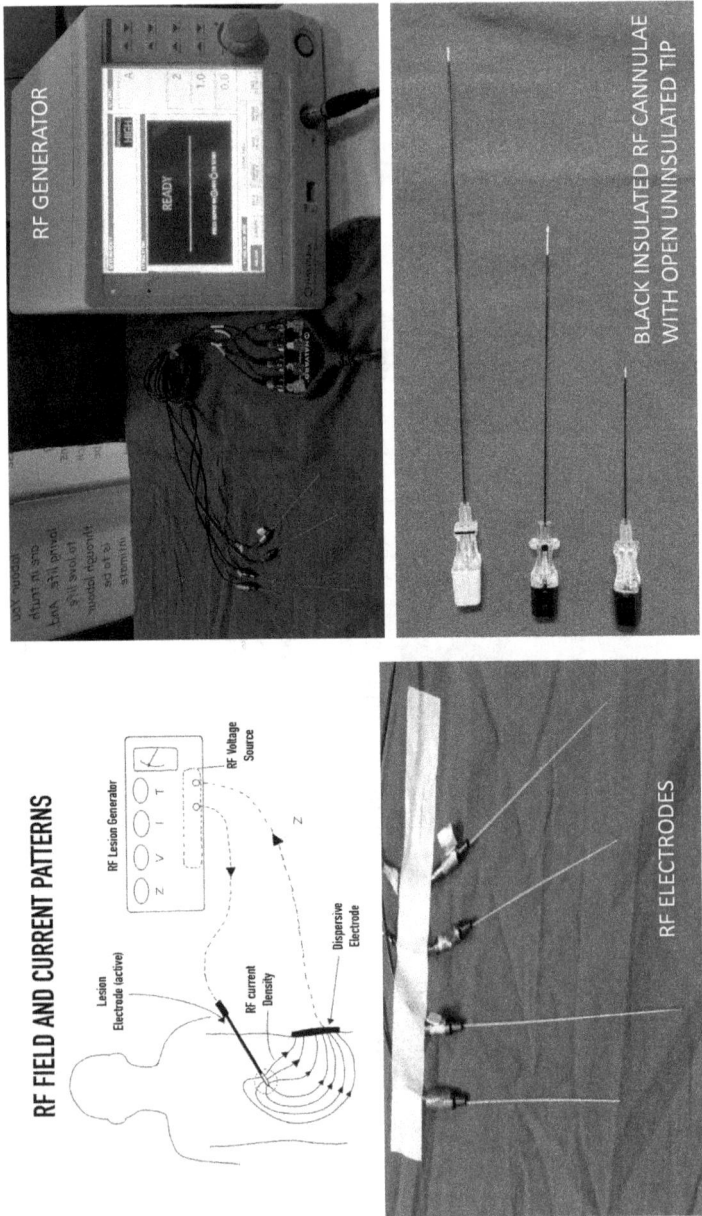

Figure 21. Top row: Diagram of radiofrequency (RF) current flow circuit and RF generator. Bottom row: Electrodes and insulated (black coated) needles with open tip.

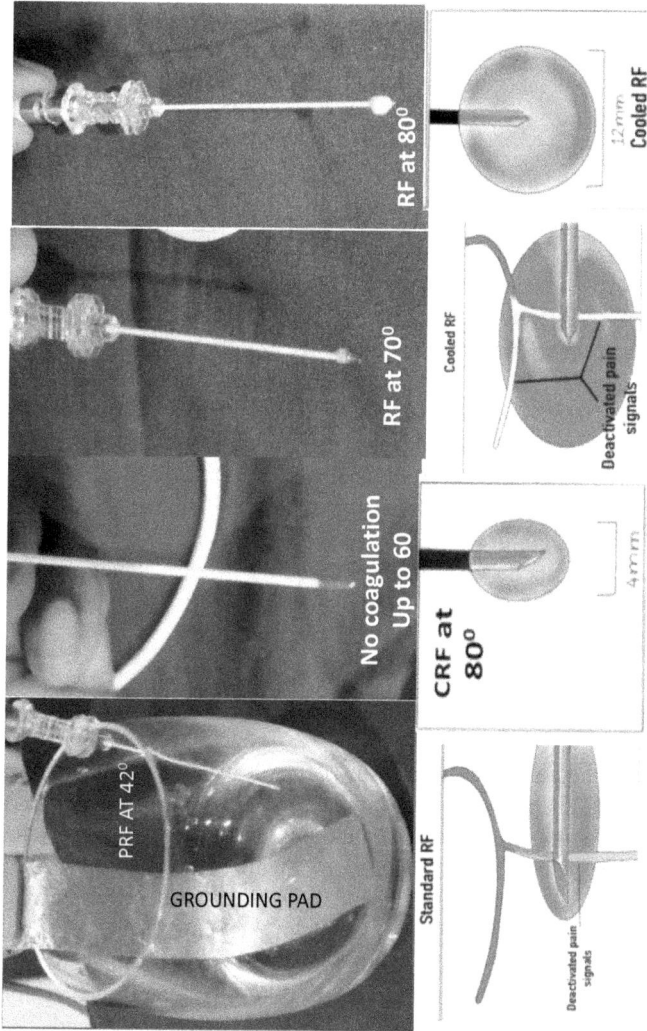

Figure 22. Top left to right: Egg white in a glass (with a grounding electrode) shows no coagulation with radiofrequency needle tip at 42 degrees for pulsed radiofrequency (PRF) and at 60degrees. Coagulum starts forming at 70degrees. At 80degrees, coagulation burn is obvious. Bottom row: 4 mm burn with conventional RF and a 12 mm burn with cooled RF.

electrical impulses thereby interrupting pain transmission. Thermal RF of the facetal nerve for intractable back pain from facet arthropathy, genicular nerves for arthritis of the knee, hip, and shoulder and trigeminal ganglion in trigeminal neuralgia (TGN) is considered justifiable. At our centre however, the genicular nerves are rarely ever burnt and never the trigeminal ganglion, the vital nerve of the face; the non-destructive, nerve-sparing pulsed radiofrequency (PRF) at 42°C of the mandibular nerve, is used instead, which supplies the masticatory muscles responsible for TGN pain followed by USGDN (reference 9 of Chapter 2).

b) *Cooled RF*: This uses a much thicker probe with a jacket around the electrode for circulating water, which acts as a heat sink while delivering greater amounts of RF energy for prolonged exposure without letting the temperature go too high and yet produces a 12 mm lesion. The 12 mm cooled RF lesion burns all branches of the genicular nerve for treating knee pain from arthritis. It is preferred to the 4 mm thermal RF lesion, which may be too small to reach the aberrant nerves or may miss smaller branches altogether (Figure 22). Given the neuromyopathy perspective, at Ashirvad, our preferred mode of RF is the nerve sparing PRF of all the nerves supplying knee muscles followed by USGDN, instead of focusing just on genicular nerves. PRF uses 22-gauge needles, which are less than half the size of the cooled RF probe and avoid creating 12 mm burns of vital tissue.

c) *Pulsed radiofrequency (PRF)*: The RF energy is delivered in short bursts or pulses to allow temperature dissipation between two pulses to hold the temperature steady at 40–42°C, ensuring there is no burn injury to the nerve (Figure 22). In knee arthritis, painful MTrPs and taut bands stiffen and restrict the free quadriceps movement with a resultant continuous pull at its tendinous insertion into the patella (kneecap) to produce inflammation (Figure 23), which expresses itself as the swollen painful knee (hallmark osteoarthritis symptom). PRF of the entire nerve supply of the knee (Figure 24) is a patient-friendly technique, which reversibly suppresses only the thinnest nerves that carry pain, to significantly relieve pain and swelling for three-to-six months. Thereafter, USGDN consistently extends the post-PRF pain relief for years by relaxing the taut bands and the MTrPs to markedly reduce the patellar pull and allowing the muscles to work better without causing inflammation. Any pain recurrence

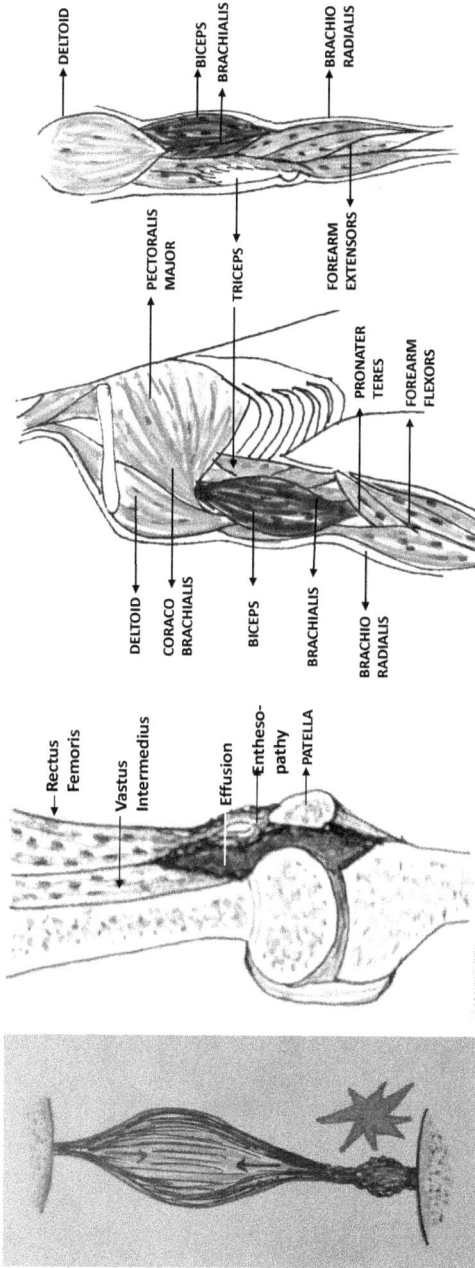

ENTHESOPATHY

EFFUSION BETWEEN RECTUS FEMORIS & VASTUS INTERMEDIUS

FRONT VIEW OF UPPER ARM MUSCLES

LATERAL VIEW OF UPPER LIMB MUSCLES

Figure 23. Left: MTrPs and taut bands pull on tendons to cause enthesopathy. Middle: MTrPs shorten the quadriceps to pull the patella (kneecap) causing painful inflammation and fluid collection around the patella in arthritis. Right: The darker painful biceps with MTrPs causes pain and compromised movement with latent MTrP formation(shown as dark spots), which triggers local twitch reflexes in all the upper limb muscles during USGDN.

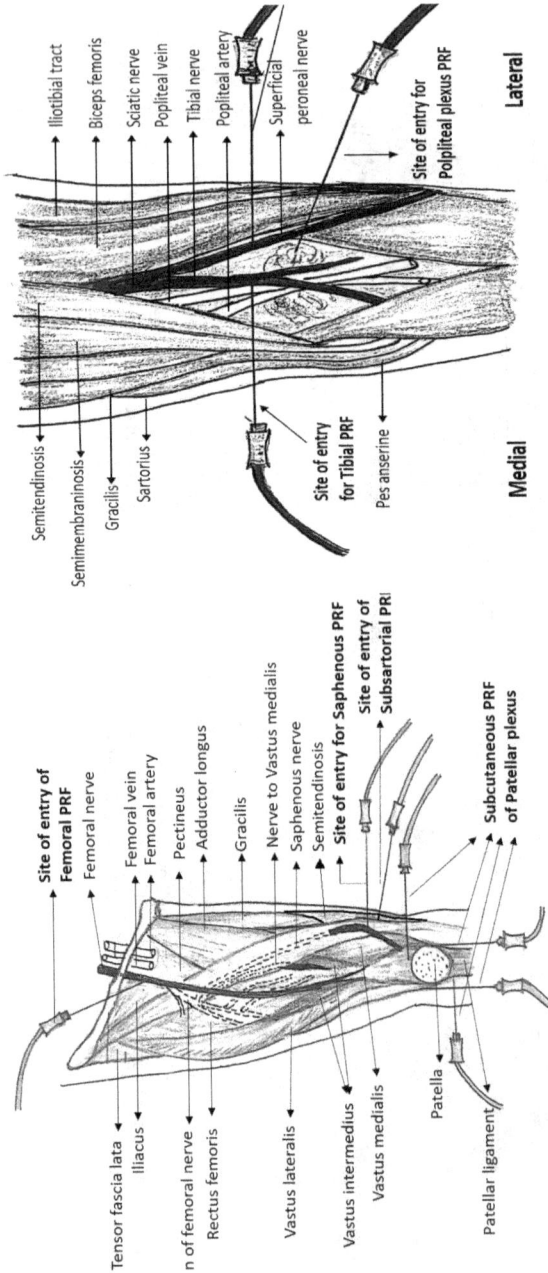

Figure 24. Anatomy of knee muscles from front and back & sites of needle introduction for PRF of knee.

triggered by activity is reliably reversed by repeated USGDNs. This empowers patients to increase their daily activities with significant, systematic, and cumulative reversal of the disability, allowing them to resume an active lifestyle. USGDN takes comprehensive cognizance of overall interactive muscle functions and the alterations of the innate muscle structure by MTrPs in various pains. For example, the stiffness from MTrPs in the biceps muscle of the arm embarrasses and stresses the upper extremity muscles, which support/oppose the biceps' actions (Figure 23). This stress leads to satellite MTrP generation and LTRs on USGDN in all these co-working muscles. This understanding has led to similar innovative PRF+USGDN combinations, which help in various chronic pain conditions like avascular necrosis (AVN) of the hip (including post-Covid AVN), frozen shoulder, migraine, trigeminal neuralgia, neuromyopathic pains after surgery, and cancer treatments.

B) *Continuous nerve blocks (CNB)*

This is a particularly effective advanced intervention identical to regional anaesthesia provided for surgeries and labour analgesia for childbirth. A very fine epidural or peripheral nerve catheter is positioned near the nerve using ultrasound and nerve stimulator guidance. It is then connected to an electrically driven or elastomeric pump where a rubber balloon stretched by local anaesthetic (LA) gradually collapses to automatically inject LA through the catheter. Since the nerves are continuously bathed in LA, the pain relief is not only instantaneous but also continuous. This is equally effective for single nerves, nerve plexuses, and the spinal cord via the epidural space (Figures 25, 26, and 27, respectively). It meaningfully resolves peripheral and spinal sensitizations yielding very good results in some very difficult pain conditions, such as failed back surgery, post-surgical pains, coccygodynia pain, PBS/ICS, chronic pelvic pains, CRPS, and recalcitrant postherpetic neuralgia (PHN).

Effective and comprehensively administered CNB requires a clear understanding of the gate control concept.[8] Any pain, which has produced spinal or central sensitization with 'windup' of pain transmission, requires a treatment that incorporates 'unwinding' of the sensitization. Since the windup results from continuous and intense bombardment of the neural gate by pain impulses travelling in the pain pathway, unwinding has to reduce the impulse barrage bombarding the neural gate (Figure 6, Chapter 1). Oral neuromodulators, analgesics, and anti-inflammatories can reduce impulse input to the spinal cord but cannot

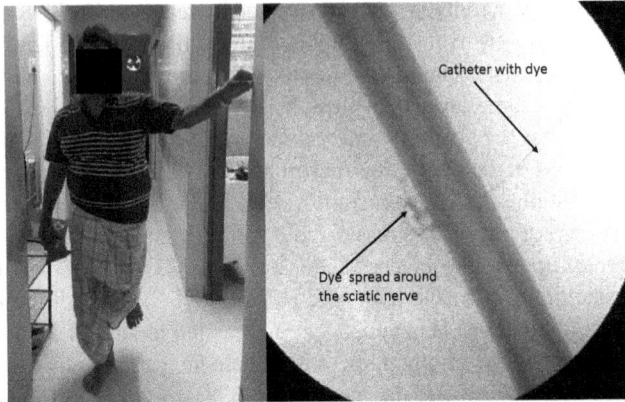

Figure 25. Left: Previously wheelchair-bound patient putting his entire weight on the CRPS right leg after 20 days of sciatic CNB from the pump in his right hand and USGDN. Right: the catheter with radio-opaque dye seen.

suppress the windup totally. CNB causes total unwinding by completely blocking the neural sodium channels and prevents the transmission of the pain impulse to the spinal cord. Epidural CNB blocks the spinal cord itself with local anaesthetic infusion. A single LA injection stops the flow of pain impulses for 2–5 hours, depending on the LA and other added drugs but a continuous LA infusion can stop pain transmission for as long as the catheter is in place. The catheter *in situ* for 5–7 days, provides a "pain holiday", which achieves a fairly significant degree of unwinding (Figures 25 to 27).

A catheter is a foreign body that breaches the skin and can act as a nidus for infection. The patient has to be on antibiotics as long as the catheter is in position. Peripheral catheter infections are less risky than those caused by epidural catheters, which have the possibility of causing meningitis, a potentially life-threatening complication. Patients are made well aware of the possible complications and risks before seeking their consent. They must be more of partners and co-contributors rather than just passive recipients of these treatments. Despite antibiotics, infections can still occur, so catheter techniques are reserved only for patients with such excruciating and crippling pains that test the patients' endurance beyond limits. Some patients experience so much pain that they feel it is not worth living. Catheter treatments work wonders for such people. We have been able to provide relief from this kind of pain to patients who have gone onto lead normal lives.

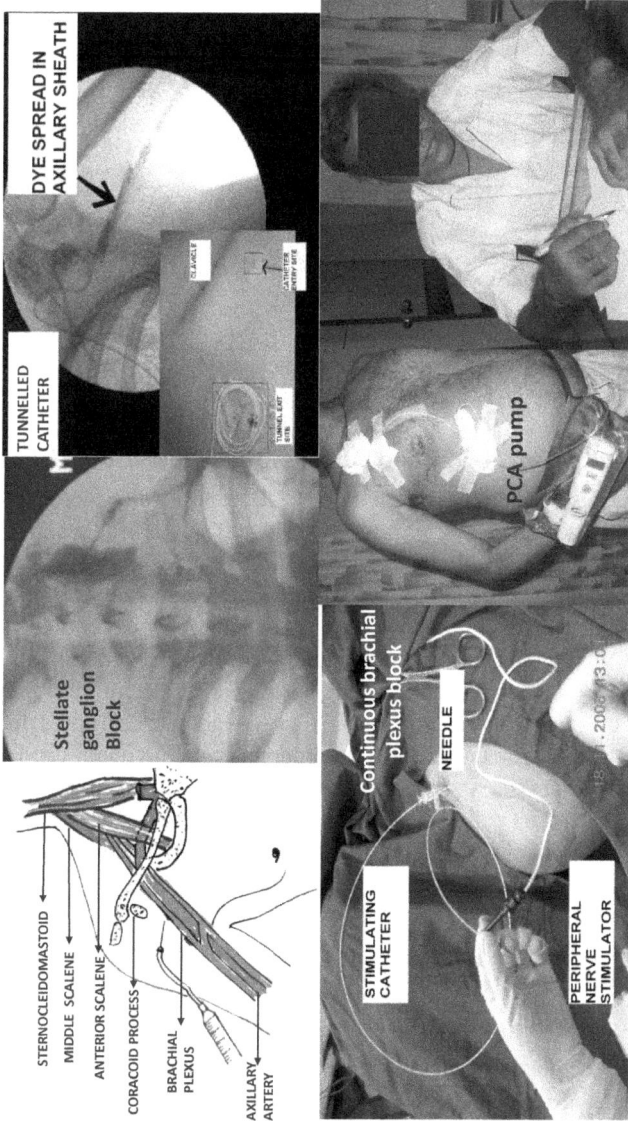

Figure 26. Top row left: Diagram of brachial plexus block. Middle and right: Stellate ganglion and brachial plexus dye spread. Inset shows the tunnelled rolled catheter. Bottom row: Continuous nerve stimulation ensures catheter proximity to the plexus. Middle: The catheter connected to a patient-controlled analgesia (PCA) pump. Writing after USGDN.

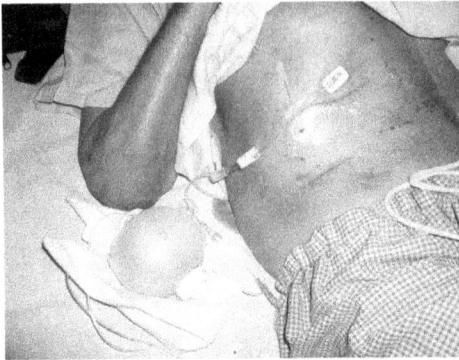

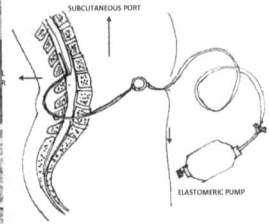

DIAGRAMMATIC REPRESENTATION
OF EPIDURAL PORT WITH
EXTERNAL PUMP

EPIDURAL CATHETER CONNECTED TO SUBCUTANEOUS PORT WITH
EXTERNAL PUMP. PORT IN SITU FOR 10 MONTHS WITH NO INFECTION

Figure 27. Epidural port and its diagrammatic representation.

C) *Intrathecal pump (ITP) or intradural drug delivery systems (IDDS)*

ITP or IDDS is a sophisticated form of CNB from a fully-implanted system. A silastic catheter is introduced through a spinal needle placed in the spinal canal into the cerebrospinal fluid (CSF). The catheter is connected through a silastic tubing to a titanium pump, implanted into the abdominal wall. The pump delivers an extremely slow continuous infusion of minute doses of morphine and/or local anaesthetic directly into the CSF, surrounding the spinal cord at a predetermined rate controlled by a microprocessor device in the pump; extra doses for unexpected surges of pain can also be programmed. The pump can be refilled through the skin, similar to the injections into a chemotherapy port (Figure 28). This is an extremely effective technique to provide excellent pain relief in terminally-ill cancer patients with uncontrolled pain, and in severely spastic conditions. The major disadvantages are firstly, the prohibitive cost of more than INR 10,00,000, making it impractical for many, and secondly, the possibility of several complications, as detailed on the Internet.

D) *Spinal cord stimulator (SCS)*

SCS is a fully implanted system. The electrode is permanently implanted in the epidural space outside the CSF and is connected to a microcurrent generator implanted into the buttock. There are many varieties of SCSs that deliver various permutations and combinations of stimulation currents either to the spinal cord (SCS) or to the dorsal root ganglion (DRG) on the sensory nerve just before it enters the spinal cord. A recent

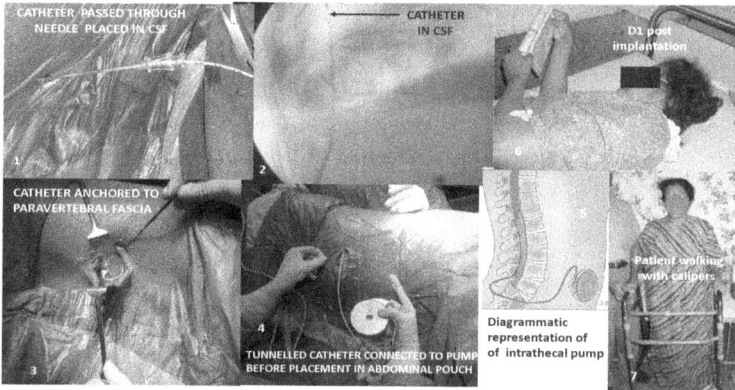

Figure 28. Intrathecal pump implantation and the resumption of normal activities post implantation.

article on the comparison of SCS with conventional medical management (CMM) on 7560 patients concluded that despite the high cost SCS did not reduce opioid dosage, nor pain injections, nor RF procedures, nor surgery.[9] After two years, one-fifth of the patients required device revision or its complete removal. This study was significant enough to merit an editorial[10] because it was an independent, large study, unfunded by SCS manufacturers. Previous SCS publications had shown benefits in controlling pain (but not disability) in CRPS and the failed back surgery syndrome but had the limitations of small patient numbers and author bias because of industry funding. The editorial concluded that improved functioning was more indicative of the treatment efficacy than just a reduction in the pain score.

Exclusive innovations

Ultrasound guided dry needling (USGDN)

USGDN distinguishes the Ashirvad approach and is based on a different understanding of the pathophysiology of chronic pains. Pain clinics across the world focus on using and developing basic or advanced procedures to address nerves, be it blocks, RF, SCS, or ITP. But experience over decades has shown:

- Nerve blocks may work well but only partially and temporarily.[3,4,11,12] Their efficacy is limited because muscles are still left out of the equation.

- Neuromodulator medications and opioids are often prescribed to cover the lacunae of nerve blocks and to augment their effect.
- Opioids are notoriously ineffective in controlling neuromyopathic pain. However, they induce a 'high' (euphoria), that definitely makes the patient happy and temporarily masks some of the pain. This makes opioids a double-edged sword; as the euphoria wanes, the pain returns with a vengeance leading to drug-seeking behaviour, dose escalation with diminishing efficacy, craving, addiction, all of which have probably contributed to the current opioid epidemic in the US.

The efficacy of USGDN in reversing neuromyopathic pain can have a far-reaching impact on the opioid crisis. However, the concept of neuromyopathy and the vital importance of muscle contribution to *all* chronic pains is yet to be acknowledged and the efficacy of USGDN in reversing or circumventing the opioid crisis is a hitherto globally unexplored possibility.

This global practice of addressing only the nerves and ignoring the muscles, which are the actual expressors of pain, is like clapping with one hand. This is because the original, basic concepts in pain management came from pioneers in orthopaedics, rheumatology, and neurology who viewed pain from their nerve-centric perspective. Pain was never the main focus of these specialties; they had to treat pain only because there was no other option. When pain management emerged as an independent specialty, anaesthesiologists automatically became pain specialists by default because of their familiarity with opioids and expertise in relieving acute surgical pain with nerve blocks. Unfortunately, chronic pain is altogether a very different 'animal' incessantly hounding hapless patients. Contemporary pain management comprises some very sophisticated interventions targeting various parts of the nervous system, based on inherited, age-old concepts, which have never been critically scrutinized nor challenged. These have, historically, been assumed to be responsible for pain. Yet many chronic pains remain untreatable enigmas. Opioids are then generously prescribed to cover the residual pains persisting after the quasi-effective neural interventions, resulting in opioid addictions.

Because the involvement of motor nerves (neuromyopathy) in causing MTrPs and MPS is neither recognized nor acknowledged, the contribution of muscles as the primary cause of pain is naturally missed. The Ashirvad protocol made the paradigm shift in the way the patient is approached, incorporating an "out-of-the-box" thought process of looking for MPS/MTrPs in *all* pains, particularly neuropathic pains. Therefore, the manner of recording histories, clinical examinations and thereafter, patient management are all different.

Most of our pain understanding, especially of the difficult types of pain, what relieves them and what does not, has come from the experience with patients and not from any book or scientific literature. In fact, in the years between 2004 and 2007 USGDN would routinely achieve clinical success that was unbelievable and inexplicable by contemporary literature. Although the success in pain relief was easy, finding explanations for the success were baffling. After working closely with patients, interacting with them, listening to their difficulties, and paying attention to their feedback about what worked and what didn't, the Gordian Knot of chronic pain began to unravel, particularly neuropathic pain. Developments and innovations of unique Ashirvad treatments to successfully relieve pain and disability in many extremely difficult conditions became possible only because of the interactive guidance from patients.

USGDN is based on a radically different understanding of chronic pain—that the muscle is the final common factor in *all* chronic pains because motor nerves are the first responders in neuropathic pains. USGDN produces an instantaneous, physical "needle effect" of immediate and complete analgesia of the pain spot independent of any drug injections (Figure 29). Thus, USGDN eliminates the root cause of MPS in most chronic pains by deactivating the MTrPs.

USGDN utilizes commercially available 32-gauge disposable, filiform solid acupuncture needles ranging between 13 and 120 mm (Figure 30). These needles are gently introduced under ultrasound visualization into the painful muscle after the skin has been numbed by local anaesthetic cream (EMLA, called Prilox in India). It cannot be emphasized enough that despite using the same tools, USGDN has nothing in common with acupuncture, which does not acknowledge muscles. Acupuncture needles are used only because they are the thinnest needles available in the market. USGDN is a highly evolved version of DN, which is another technique used by physiotherapists around the world to relieve MPS pain. DN targets only the obviously painful point (presumed MTrP) in one muscle while USGDN targets all coworking muscles to restore functionality and in the process, automatically relieves pain. The differences between acupuncture, simple dry needling, and USGDN are shown in Table 1.

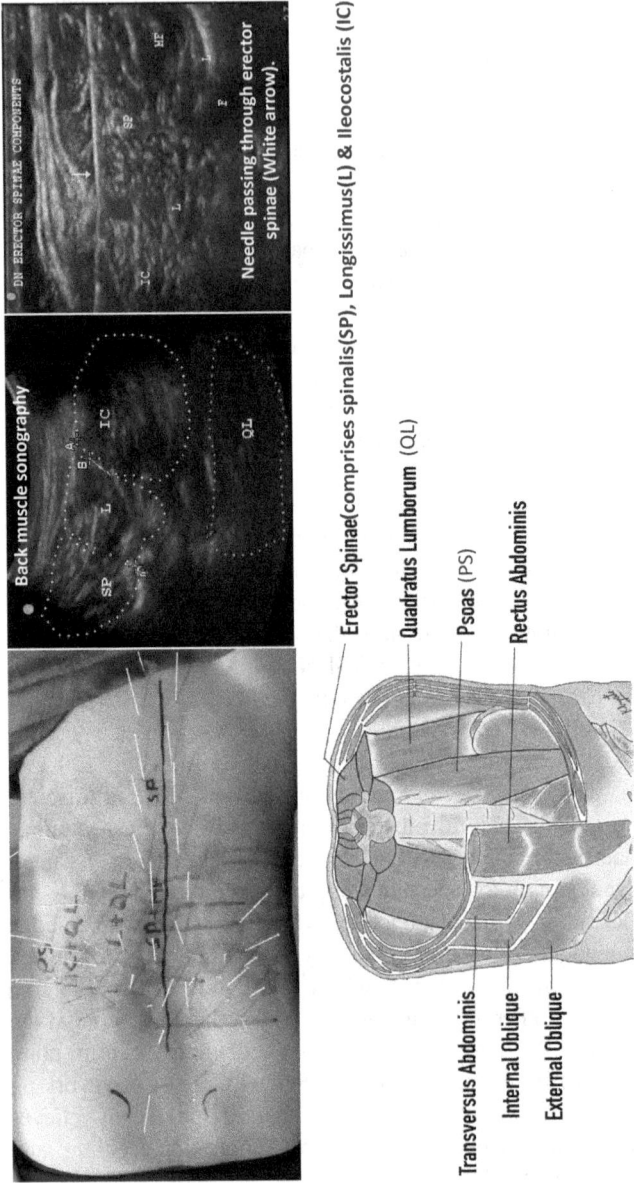

Figure 29. Top left: USGDN targets spinalis (SP), and multifidus (MF), the longissimus (L) and the deeper quadratus lumborum. The outermost needles (PS) travel through the iliocostalis (IC) to the psoas muscle. Bottom: diagram of the back muscles.

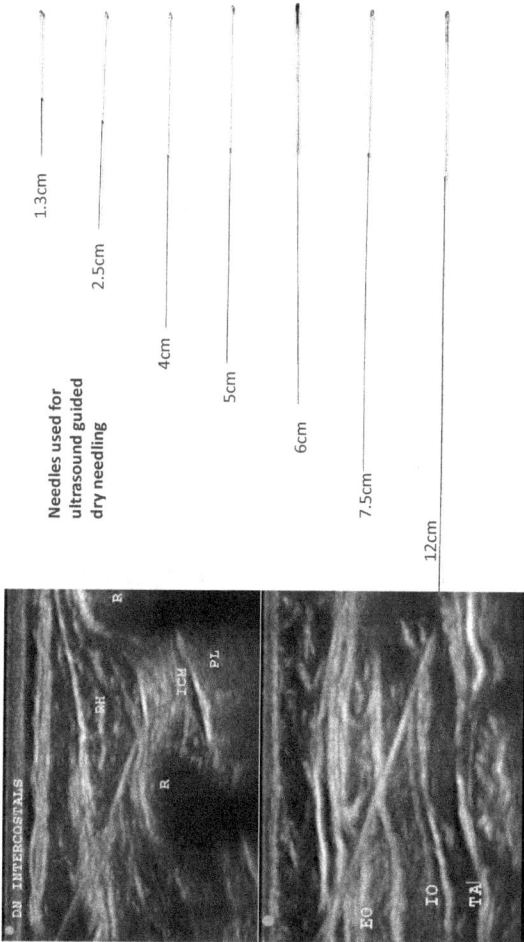

Figure 30. Top left: Needle in rhomboid (RH) and intercostal muscle (ICM). Bottom left: Needle in external oblique (EO), Internal oblique (IO), and transversus abdominis (TA) muscles. Whole needle visualization avoids pleural (PL) and peritoneal injury. Rib (R). Right: Needles used for USGDN.

Table 1. Salient differences between acupuncture, conventional DN and USGDN.[13]

	Acupuncture	Conventional simple DN	USGDN
Diagnostic process	Solely based on Chinese philosophy	Physical demonstration of MTrPs necessary for diagnosis of myofascial pain.	History and examination by a pain physician necessary for the medical diagnosis of neuropathy and/or myofascial pain.
Physical examination for MTrPs	No concept of MTrP	Physical examination to find the most painful points for needle insertion mandatory	Physical examination to determine the painful muscles to be needled + Ultrasound examination mandatory
Needle insertion	Blind insertion into specific acupoints located on meridians	Needles inserted blindly into the most painful part of muscles demonstrated by clinical exam and into palpable taut bands.	Needle insertion under ultrasound visualization into all the muscles underlying the area indicated in the pain diagram and its co-workers
Number of needles/ session	6–10 (more used occasionally)	6–10 needles per session	30–60 needles per session
Needle length	13–25 mm	25–50 mm	13 mm–120 mm
Duration of needle *in situ* maintenance	Usually, 20 minutes	< 1 min. Needle is introduced, pumped up & down and withdrawn, all in a few seconds.	20–30 minutes. The needle is slowly advanced in small increments, and when at maximum depth, left *in situ* or for 20–30 minutes."
No of sessions	Not specified	Up to 6 sessions.	10–12 sessions but may go up to 20 sessions.
Sequence of events on needle insertion	Not anticipated nor looked for	Needles introduced only into maximally painful areas and taut bands. Muscle jumps (local twitch reflex or LTR) elicited by pumping the needle up and down multiple times.	Needles introduced not just into the maximally painful areas but into several points in the whole muscle with no attempts to elicit LTRs. But ultrasound routinely visualized multiple LTRs in co-working muscles and in areas of muscle where physical exam does not detect MTrPs.

Practitioner Expertise	Muscle anatomy not needed	Knowledge of muscle anatomy necessary.	In-depth knowledge of muscle anatomy, sono-anatomy, and the ability to steer needles under ultrasound are essential.
Associated risks and complications	Neurovascular & visceral injuries Reported	Blind procedure with visceral and neurovascular injuries reported. Bruising common.	Ultrasound visualization *avoids* the risk of visceral and neurovascular injuries. Bruising commonly seen.
Indications	For pain and many painless diseases	Only indicated for pain	Mainly indicated for Pain. But also, for movement disorders, cerebral palsy, deformities after stroke, vertigo, hiccups.

** Needles are left *in situ* for 20–30 minutes during USGDN because ultrasound videos have shown LTR activity persisting for about 15–20 minutes, and rarely, even 40 minutes, indicating that longer maintenance is required to end the LTR and deactivate the MTrP. While the LTR is ongoing, the muscle grips the needle, making withdrawal difficult and painful. After the LTR subsides, the muscle relaxes, and the needle comes out smoothly and painlessly and patients report reduction in pain.

Evolution of simple DN into the USGDN

USGDN emerged from DN as a game changer to become an integral and unique pillar of pain management at Ashirvad. Twenty years ago, nerve blocks and RF procedures performed accurately with attention to the minutest detail produced pain relief but that would last only a few days or weeks and the pain would return in full force after some unguarded movement or exertion. It was extremely disheartening (and puzzling). Obviously, the key factor causing unaddressed pain was being missed making the patients return. Thus started the search for the missing link in pain management. It was consistently found that the patients had MPS with tender rope-like bands in their muscles, which could be rolled between the fingers. Instead of dismissing this as an unrelated or secondary issue due to muscle disuse and prescribing opioids (which were anyway difficult to obtain at that time in India), these patients were treated with a more extensive version of the IMS/DN practiced by physiotherapists. Surprisingly, after six to eight sessions of this extensive DN, patients not only reported sustained pain relief but also the ability to adopt a more active lifestyle. Although these unexpectedly, good results were exhilarating they were also puzzling because these results came after addressing muscles which are usually dismissed in pain literature as secondary, "also ran" pain generators.

Why had other erudite pain specialists across the world, who had written books and monographs on pain, not referred to muscles in any pain condition? Especially, in backache patients with intervertebral disc prolapse and facet arthritis, who were returning with pain recurrence after a block-induced short respite? Why were the patients doing so much better once USGDN was introduced after having failed the blocks? Nevertheless, the results were 100 per cent obvious, that with USGDN, disabled and bedridden patients were resuming a normal life.

Alternately, was this something that was too basic to be considered significant by the pain management community? What sustained a continued search for answers with retained objectivity, was the 20 years' experience in a difficult and complex branch like paediatric anaesthesia where textbooks had changed as science and technology evolved, as new information got verified and validated. Therefore, it was logical to expect that such *de novo* information would take time to be further verified and validated.

It was clear that a better understanding of muscle anatomy was mandatory to understand these results. Therefore, it was necessary to return to the medical drawing-board in the cadaver lab. Relearning muscle anatomy, with far greater focus, confirmed how essential the complete knowledge of muscles is to meaningfully understand chronic pain in general, and MPS in particular. The comprehensive understanding of muscle anatomy and interpretation of muscle action made it clear that pain and functional impairment are two sides of the same pathology. Functional impairment is not just because of pain but is an independent manifestation of muscle problems in executing daily functions. After continuously observing patients with various types of pain and their response to USGDN, it became obvious that the pain and tenderness at one MTrP is just the tip of the iceberg. The actual pathology lies deeper in the multitudes of MTrPs (both active and latent) scattered across not just the entire muscle but also its functional counterparts because of the interdependent complexity of the muscle function (Figure 23). This radically changed the approach to DN by going beyond addressing only the demonstrable MTrP at the most painful area in isolation (as in simple DN) towards addressing the entire muscle harbouring the demonstrable MTrP, and the co-working muscle groups. This was based on the presumption that when patients complain of pain, the actual cause (MTrP) is in the muscles underlying the painful area (Figures 8, 9, 29–31a,b) and their agonists and antagonists. Additional MTrPs present in all these muscles have to be decisively reversed by USGDN. This understanding has been consistently confirmed by musculoskeletal ultrasonography (MSKUSG) in the past 18 years by the ultrasound visualization of multitudes of LTRs in coworking muscles during USGDN. A normal muscle does not react to needle introduction with LTR, which is an exclusive indicator of a MTrP. LTRs are routinely seen in seemingly normal and painless co-workers of a painful muscle. Thus, in a single session of dry needling, the agonist, antagonist, synergists, and fixator muscles are collectively addressed with at least three to four needles per muscle, using 40 to 50 needles per session. Every pain has a MTrP distribution pattern in many muscle groups as shown by ultrasound visualization of the sequence of events in the muscle on needle introduction. This understanding of 18 years ago, that muscles form the warp and weft of the pain fabric has been regularly and repeatedly re-confirmed. This understanding has made USGDN of various pains and their variegated presentations, very comprehensive

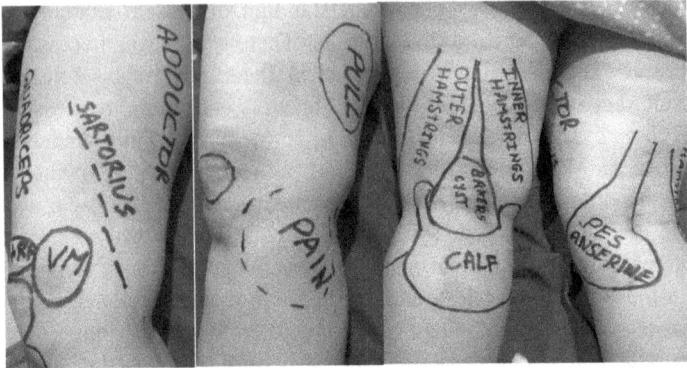

knee pain areas due to sartorius, adductors, inner hamstrings, vastus medius spasms

Figure 31a. The pain referral patterns of the inner and back of thigh muscles affected in knee and facet arthritis or sciatica.

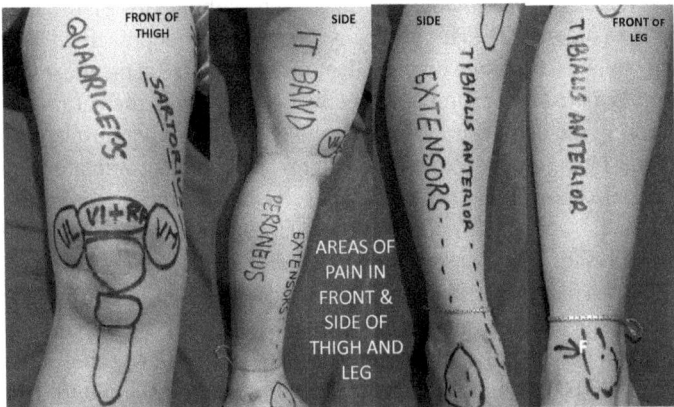

Figure 31b. The pain referral patterns of anterior thigh and anterolateral leg muscles in sciatica, knee arthritis, and other pains.

with routine reversal of all kinds of common and uncommon, "difficult-to-treat" pain conditions (Table 2). The combination of target-specific USGDN and ultrasound guided Botox, coupled with neural interventions achieves up to 50–60 per cent relief within the first two weeks. Table 3 shows a snapshot of the results achieved in patient subsets from a set of 12,000 patients.

Table 2. Some common and uncommon pains successfully reversed at Ashirvad.

Locomotor pains	Chronic post-surgery pain	Neuropathic pains	Neuralgias	CRPS Type 1
Back pain and sciatica, from various causes	Back surgery	Post-stroke pains	Trigeminal	
Osteoarthritic knee and hip pain, rheumatoid arthritis	Knee and hip surgery	Cancer	Glosso-Pharyngeal	**CRPS Type 2 or Causalgia**
Neck and upper extremity pain from various causes	Abdominal surgery	Central pain	Occipital	
Frozen shoulder pain, tennis, and golfer's elbow	Thoracic surgery	Phantom pain	Herpes, post herpetic neuralgia	
Carpal tunnel pain syndrome	Even craniotomy	Migraine, facial pains		
Ankylosing spondylitis	Facial surgery	Endometriosis		Writer's cramp
Other Sero+ve & Sero-ve arthropathy	Cancer surgery	Chronic pelvic pain		
Lower extremity pains	Post-ENT surgery	Post-radiation and post chemotherapy pain		

USGDN, either as a sole modality or as an adjuvant to neural interventions, is a simple, yet safe technique in pain management. It dramatically alters the outcomes of interventional pain management, by automatically and simultaneously addressing both the disability and pain by targeting muscles. Hence, it could tackle the western opioid epidemic by reducing the need for opioids. Ultrasound allows seeing the whole length of the needle in real time (Figures 29, 30) and demonstrates many hitherto undescribed muscle events during USGDN. The uncovering of so many facts, presently unknown to science, has developed an alternative understanding of pain that is poised to rewrite the practice of pain management world-wide.

Ultrasound guided Botox

This has developed as an extremely useful offshoot of USGDN where the Botox doses and the muscles to be injected, are determined by

Table 3. A snapshot of subsets of chronic pains in 12,000 patients treated from 2004 to 2019.[13]

Conditions	No.	Brief synopsis of the number of patients benefited and the extent of benefit
Neuropathic pains	1221	> 90% achieved end point of meaningful and lasting pain relief with PRF + USGDN with Botox/trigger point injections – suggestive of neuromyopathic pains
CRPS Types 1 & 2	220	End point of 100% pain relief and 90% disability relief; return to work in > 95% achieved within 45 days with USGDN as the main treatment. Forty patients received continuous brachial plexus block. (See Chapter 5 section 1)
Post-spine injury (old terminology-causalgia)	3	*All* patients had pain resolution with lumbar sympathetic PRF and USGDN. One with high velocity rifle shot injury has no pain, walks with callipers and creates a national record in pistol shooting. He returns to a desk job in the special forces of Indian army. Others after traffic accidents are pain-free and have resumed their professional activities.
Brachial plexus injuries (BPI)	11	Ten had complete pain relief with USGDN indicating pain in BPI was myofascial. Five regained movements (DASH scores improved by 30–40%) raising the query whether USGDN relieved the low-grade agonist/antagonist co-contraction causing the motor deficit.
Post-stroke pains	12	Eight had > 80% pain relief after three USGDN sessions and motor improvement after 10–12 USGDN sessions. Three received ultrasound-guided Botox injection into muscles for rapid pain relief. Four post-stroke CRPS were reversed.
Deafferentation pains	2	One became pain free with only USGDN and the other with a combination of baclofen intrathecal pump for her spasms and USGDN for motor improvement.
Phantom pains	3	One paediatric patient and two adults reported a distinct reduction of the frequency, duration, and intensity of phantom pains. One adult requires maintenance USGDN (2–3 sessions) once in 3–6 months.
Herpes, post herpetic neuralgia	35	> 90% achieved reduction of hyperaesthesia, allodynia and pain with three USGDN sessions and complete, lasting relief with 10–12 sessions with no later recurrences. Five also received local intercostal nerve PRF.

Table 3 contd. ...

...Table 3 contd.

Conditions	No.	Brief synopsis of the number of patients benefited and the extent of benefit
Trigeminal neuralgia	44	*All* patients reached the end point of remission with complete pain relief with USGDN of the masticatory and neck muscles. Fourteen patients with frequent pains (> 6 VAS) received PRF of the mandibular nerve. End point of no medications achieved in > 80%. Rest required minimal carbamazepine to maintain remission. Two patients opted for surgery while in remission.
Post-surgical neuropathic pains	> 86	> 90% patients achieved end point of pain relief and improved functionality with USGDN alone, strongly suggesting neuromyopathy. Some required local blocks or PRF, local and general strengthening exercises. They could stop/reduce opioids.
Failed back surgery	102	> 70% of patients reached the end point of pain relief, stop/reduce opioids, neuromodulators with USGDN+ neural intervention. They improved their daily activities and resumed active professional life.
Back pain from various causes	809	> 85% of patients reached the end point pain relief, resuming active professional life and stop/reduce opioids, neuromodulators with USGDN+neural interventions.
Knee pain from Osteoarthritis	396	> 95% of patients achieved end points like, pain relief, improved functionality, stopped/reduced opioids, neuromodulators. USGDN with or without PRF showed consistent predictable and meaningful improvement of daily activities and resumption of active life.
Knee pain from rheumatoid arthritis (RA)	10	*All* patients achieved end point of pain relief, could stop/reduce opioids, neuromodulators but with continued RA treatment. Combination of USGDN+PRF showed consistent predictable, dramatic improvement of pain, and quality of life (SF16), with hitherto impossible active lifestyles.
Frozen shoulder	110	> 85% of patients achieved end point of pain relief, stop/reduce analgesics. USGDN +PRF of the composite nerve supply of all the shoulder muscles allowed a sustained, painless return of all shoulder movements within 30–45 days.
Headaches and migraine	81	> 95% patients achieved end point of pain relief with USGDN+USG guided Botox into all the neck and suboccipital triangle muscles. C1–C3 PRF was done in selected patients. The frequency and the severity of attacks and medications reduction > 90%

Table 3 contd. ...

...Table 3 contd.

Conditions	No.	Brief synopsis of the number of patients benefited and the extent of benefit
Chronic pelvic pain (21)	35	> 85% achieved the end point of meaningful pain relief, improved urinary/rectal function, improved quality of life (SF16), could stop/reduce opioids, neuromodulators after combination therapy with continuous caudal block, Botox and USGDN of pelvic floor muscles in this difficult pain condition.
Myofascial pains	247	*All* patients achieved the end point of pain relief, could stop/reduce analgesics while increasing activities. USGDN, Botox/trigger point injections ± PRF of nerves to local muscles allowed a sustained, painless return to higher activity levels with physiotherapy.
Writer's cramp	6	*All* had complete pain relief from pain after 8–10 sessions of USGDN.
Fibromyalgia	11	> 60% had relief of their pain BUT pains came up elsewhere. They could reduce analgesics but any increase in activities caused pain recurrence necessitating medication increase. Eventually combination of USGDN with Botox/trigger point injections/PRF of nerves to local muscles allowed a better quality of life on SF16. The end point of lasting pain relief was not possible, but USGDN made a big difference as a supportive therapy.
Cancer pain	94	Neuropathic pains after cancer and its therapies are majorly neuromyopathic and respond to opioid sparing effects of neural blocks+ USGDN and USGDN guided Botox. They all achieved end point of a good quality of life with pains < 1–2 with minimum opioids.

the USGDN findings; resistance offered to needle passage and LTR visualization. USGDN + Botox protocols work symbiotically:

1. A Botox injection reduces the pain associated with a subsequent USGDN procedure, making it indispensable for patients with needle phobia.

2. One session of Botox produces an effect similar to six-to-eight sessions of USGDN, hence cuts short the treatment time for outstation patients with tight time schedules.

3. Conversely, USGDN optimizes and fine tunes Botox effects; the MTrPs and taut bands left unaddressed by the low dose Botox get

eliminated within 4–5 USGDN sessions, adding tremendous value to Botox efficacy.

4. Botox + USGDN form two aspects of a personalized treatment that can be stand-alone or in addition to neural interventions.

5. Invaluable for terminally-ill patients, who need quick effects to optimize their precious time.

6. Quick relief from Botox can be life changing for extremely despondent or suicidal patients.

7. Post Botox USGDN helps patients who have failed to get relief after repeated Botox for dystonia and migraine treatments earlier (see Chapter 4).

References

[1] Ryan S. D'Souza, Brendan Langford, Rachel E. Wilson, Yeng F. Her, Justin Schappell, Jennifer S. Eller, Timothy C. Evans and Jonathan M. Hagedorn. 2022. The state-of-the-art pharmacotherapeutic options for the treatment of chronic non-cancer pain. Expert Opinion on Pharmacotherapy, 23:7, 775–789, DOI: 10.1080/14656566.2022.2060741.

[2] Marris, D., Theophanous, K., Cabezon, P., Dunlap, Z. and Donaldson, M. (2021). The impact of combining pain education strategies with physical therapy interventions for patients with chronic pain: A systematic review and meta-analysis of randomized controlled trials. Physiotherapy Theory and Practice. Apr 3; 37(4): 461–72.

[3] Manchikanti, L., Sanapati, M.R., Pampati, V., Boswell, M.V., Kaye, A.D. and Hirsch, J.A. (2019). Update on reversal and decline of growth of utilization of interventional techniques in managing chronic pain in the Medicare population from 2000 to 2018. Pain Physician. 22(6): 521.

[4] Manchikanti, L., Singh, V., Kaye, A.D. and Hirsch, J.A. (2020). Lessons for better pain management in the future: Learning from the past. Pain and Therapy. 9: 373–91.

[5] Walsh, T, Malhotra, R. and Sharma, M. (2022). Radiofrequency techniques for chronic pain. BJA Education. Dec 1; 22(12): 474–83.

[6] Mahawar, B., Kannan, A., Mahawar, V. and Srinivasan, S. (2023). Intrathecal pain pumps in pain relief. Clinical Radiology. Apr 1; 78(4): 240–4.

[7] Deer, T.R., Grider, J.S., Lamer, T.J., Pope, J.E., Falowski, S., Hunter, C.W., Provenzano, D.A., Slavin, K.V., Russo, M., Carayannopoulos, A. and Shah, J.M. (2020). A systematic literature review of spine neurostimulation therapies for the treatment of pain. Pain Medicine. Jul 1; 21(7): 1421–32.

[8] Melzack, R. and Wall, P.D. (1965). Pain mechanisms: A new theory. Science. 150(699): 971–979. [PubMed:5320816].

[9] Dhruva, S.S., J. Murillo, O. Ameli et al. 2023. Long-term outcomes in use of opioids, nonpharmacologic pain interventions, and total costs of spinal cord stimulators compared with conventional medical therapy for chronic pain. JAMA Neurology. Jan 1; 80(1): 18–29.

[10] Shirvalkar, P. and L. Poree. 2023. How SAFE is real-world use of spinal cord stimulation therapy for chronic pain? JAMA Neurology. Jan 1; 80(1): 10–11.

[11] Juch, J.N., E.T. Maas, R.W. Ostelo et al. 2017. Effect of radiofrequency denervation on pain intensity among patients with chronic low back pain: the mint randomized clinical trials. Jama. Jul 4; 318(1): 68–81.

[12] Manchikanti, L., A. Soin, D.P. Mann et al. 2017. Reversal of growth of utilization of interventional techniques in managing chronic pain in Medicare population post Affordable Care Act. Pain Physician 20(7): 551.

[13] Vas, L.C. 2022. Ultrasound guided dry needling: Relevance in chronic pain. J. Postgrad. Med. Jan 1; 68(1): 1.

Chapter 4

The Ultrasound Guided Botulinum Toxin

Botulinum toxin, a neurotoxin produced by *Clostridium botulinum* bacteria gained notoriety as the cause of botulism, a dangerous form of food poisoning. In 1897, three out of 34 Belgian musicians developed gastrointestinal symptoms after consuming smoked ham at a funeral, and died. The remaining ham and the organs from the deceased showed the bacteria called *Clostridium* (spindle-shape) *botulinum* after *botulus* (Latin for sausage).[1] The toxin was isolated around 1945. In 1965, Drachman[2] demonstrated paralysis and atrophy of chicks' muscles after a botulinum toxin injection. Scott, an ophthalmologist, used it to correct squints, and was eventually approved by the US FDA in 1989 for treating squint disorders, blepharospasm (abnormal contraction of the eyelid muscles), and hemifacial spasm (involuntary spasms of half the face including the eyelid). Botulinum toxin (botox) was approved later for cervical dystonia (CD), hyperactive bladder, sialorrhea (excessive salivation), hyperhidrosis (excessive sweating), migraine, and spasticity.[3]

Botox prevents the release of the neurotransmitter acetylcholine from the nerve endings at the neuromuscular junction to cause temporary/partial paralysis. Eight distinct serotypes (A, B, C1, C2, D, E, F, and G) have been identified.[4, 5] Types A and B have been extensively studied in movement disorders in neurology, anti-aging medicine, and in pain medicine.[6, 7] Judicious use of this wonder toxin in beauty and cosmetology earned it the reputation of a "miracle toxin".

Botox for dystonia

Dystonia is a lifelong problem of uncontrolled, often painful, muscle movements (spasms). It can, at best, be given temporary limited symptomatic relief with botox injection. The botox injection is effective for 4–6 months, and needs to be repeated for relief.

Our first dystonia patient was referred for treatment of neck pain associated with dystonia because the patient could not afford botox for dystonia treatment. The patient was wincing with pain and had to stabilize his neck with his hands to prevent the involuntary side-to-side movements. USGDN was done to relieve his pain, but the interesting finding was that the dystonic movements decreased as well! Unusual results were routine in the early days of the learning process with USGDN in various pain conditions. Success came first and then the whys and hows of the unexpected success had to be elucidated, rather like reaching from behind the head to touch the nose! The surmise in this case, was that the numerous MTrPs in both the agonist and antagonist muscles of every neck movement were not only causing the pain but had also shortened the muscle fibres into taut bands, which were apparently getting stimulated with the smallest neck movements. Once initiated, the muscle irritability sustained the momentum of the movements resulting in dystonia. By relaxing both groups of muscles, systematic USGDN was apparently restoring the normal phenomenon called reciprocal inhibition, which makes the antagonist relax when the agonist contracts, and vice versa. This relaxation reduced the dystonic movements. Thereafter, regular stretching exercises of the neck muscles, helped to maintain muscle elasticity and normalcy restored by USGDN. At that time, this was an exciting revelation because it meant that dystonia, with or without pain, was treatable with USGDN!

The patient had a peculiar sitting posture, almost as if he was sliding down in the chair and was incapable of sitting straight. Apparently cervical dystonia was but a manifestation of many other major postural issues starting from his legs, up his back, and to his neck. After all, the back and torso rest on the pillars of two legs. The leg muscles in the calves and shins stabilize the knees and ankles, while the powerful thigh muscles stabilize the back and the entire body in the erect posture. He readily agreed for USGDN of his legs and back although he had no obvious symptoms there, because he was so happy to be free of pain and dystonia. His posture improved dramatically, and he was sitting upright without support, an impossible feat for him for years. He followed up for six months without any recurrences.

Thus, came the understanding that cervical dystonia involves all the layers of the neck muscles that move the neck and not just the designated culprits like sternocleidomastoid and splenius muscles. The inference was that for dystonia reversal, all the postural muscles of the legs and lower back also need to be addressed.

The next dystonia patient was someone who had experienced a failure in botox injection treatment. Systemic USGDN of the neck helped reverse the dystonia, thus re-affirming that all the neck muscles have to be addressed rather than just the sternocleidomastoid/splenius combination.

By this time, low-dose botox was being used at Ashirvad in several pain conditions in combination with neural procedures like epidural injections and PRF, to produce very good results in a short time. These experiences reiterated that one session of a low-dose botox produced an effect similar to the cumulative effect of six-to-eight sessions of USGDN, markedly reducing the treatment time, along with stiffness and pain in the muscles at rest and on movement. Additionally, an advance dose of botox significantly reduced the USGDN pain. However, two-to-three sessions of the post-botox USGDN seemed to enhance the botox effect by successfully releasing the residual taut bands left unaddressed by the low-dose of botox. All these results were uniform, across many pain conditions.

Then came another patient with recalcitrant dystonia. The contrast between his sharp, alert face and his slouched posture, with a hand on his cheek was striking. Examination revealed that he slouched because he could not sit upright and he had to firmly support his cheek to prevent the dystonic lashing of his neck from side-to-side. He had received repeated botox injections with progressively diminishing efficacy and increasing frequency till it had become totally ineffective. As the CEO of a large company, he had to address groups of people, often sitting in a chair without back support. The dystonic movements while standing and the slouch while sitting had made things very difficult for him. He quickly grasped the logic of our protocol of fine-tuning the botox effect with USGDN, the need to address the back and leg muscles because these, in turn, influence the neck muscles and the need for a PRF procedure for the nerve supply of the dystonic muscles. Ultrasound guided botox for the various muscle layers of his neck was administered. Three days later his dystonic movements had already reduced, but after the PRF of the neck nerves and four more sessions of USGDN, the dystonia ceased altogether. He spoke confidently at a conference that week that he had been dreading! However, he was still slouching while sitting without support. Therefore, his lower back and lower limb muscles were addressed next with additional ultrasound guided botox followed by systematic twice-a-week USGDN till all his problems were resolved. Interestingly, he found some dystonia institute in California, which advocated certain yoga stretches and particularly, *Chandra namaskar* (Moon salutation), as a part of dystonia therapy. *Chandra namaskar* definitely is a scientific exercise for sideway stretches to the body and perfectly complements *Surya namaskar* (Sun salutation shown later in Figure 45), which stretches the body front to back. He was already doing *Surya namaskar* as advised, and he added *Chandra namaskar* to his daily routine. He needed three more sessions of botox in the next two years. The curious coincidence was that he would have a viral fever just before the dystonia resurfaced. This was not surprising because viral fevers cause myositis (muscle inflammation), which can worsen pre-existing myofascial problems which have gone into remission after USGDN. Myositis is the reason for the pains after chikungunya infection, and in recent times, the post-covid pains and long-covid symptoms of brain fog. He was cautioned that whenever he got a viral fever he must resume the exercises or massage as soon as possible, and have a USGDN session if necessary, to ensure that the symptoms did not worsen or escalate. After three years, he did not need any treatment and continues to be dystonia-free, maintaining a good posture and an active lifestyle.

USGDN to the rescue after botox failure: A patient, whose hemifacial spasms had worsened after a botox injection, admisnistered elsewhere presented with constant facial contortions which appeared as if she was making grotesque faces. Understandably, she was very anxious, despondent, and wary. She readily agreed for USGDN after she understood the logic of fine-tuning botox effects with USGDN, and the need to address both sides of her face to restore and maintain the symmetry of the face. Within two-three sessions the frequency and severity of the spasms and the related pain decreased; as the treatment progressed, normalcy of her face was restored. She did remarkably well thereafter without any spasm or pain recurrence.

Diminishing utility of botox in migraine

Many migraine patients seek help when botox effects decrease with repeated injections. Ultrasound makes it possible to use very low doses of additional botox to be properly distributed into various neck muscles, arranged in intricate layers. Nerves that supply the neck muscles pass through the very same muscles that they supply, and their entrapment worsens the muscle spasm. When botox is followed by very precise USGDN of the complex layers of the neck muscles, particularly the LTR producing muscles, it further fine-tunes the botox effects.

Botox and back pain

Severe pulling pains in leg and thigh muscles, is a feature of intervertebral disc prolapse. These pains persist even after epidural steroid injections and are visible as resting muscles twitches on ultrasonography, Patients respond to USGDN, twice weekly, over 1 to 2 months. The ultrasound guided botox injection remarkably hastens recovery from the crippling back and leg pains within three-to-four days. Thereafter, USGDN effectively fine-tunes the botox effects so that they resume their normal personal, professional, and social activities.

A patient came to us four months after the pain from a disc prolapse failed to improve after bedrest and medical management as advised by the spine surgeon and physiotherapy at a widely advertised physiotherapy chain. A ten minutes' walk exacerbated his pain, heaviness, tingling, and numbness in the back and lower limb. He was fed-up of these limitations and enforced bedrest for most of the time.

A repeat MRI showed worsening of the disc, indicating surgery. Although he had consulted a spine surgeon, he wished to avoid surgery. This added multiple responsibilities: reducing the pain, correcting his disabilities, and most importantly, enabling him to safely avoid surgery. Treatment began with an epidural steroid injection to reduce the inflammation around the spinal nerve compressed by the disc. Botox was administered to relax the spinal muscles, which were crunching the vertebrae together forcing the disc out. The botox proved to be the ideal choice because all the muscles were not only stiff but also extremely painful, limiting the number of needles during USGDN. But one week later he had no backache or leg pain and could walk comfortably for 15 minutes at a stretch. However, he still experienced some shocks and

JUNE 2022   OCT 2022   MAY 2023

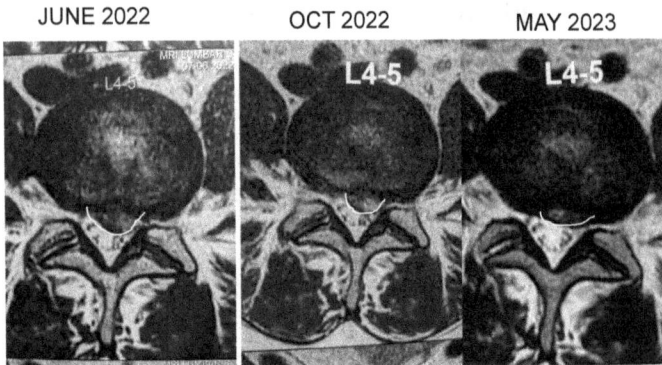

Figure 32. MRI shows prolapsed disc (left). The middle image after treatment with epidural steroid+Botox+USGDN, shows a smaller disc outline (white) with a narrower base. The lighter shade indicates a probable dissolution of prolapse by natural body scavengers. The right image 1 year later shoows an obvious reduction of disc size.

tingling in his feet, which coincided with visible LTRs in the hamstrings, adductors of the thigh, and particularly the tibialis posterior muscle. Additional botox into all these muscles and thorough systematic USGDN under temporary sciatic nerve block, relieved the tingling. Thereafter, he improved steadily, could walk 45 to 60 minutes at a stretch, climb two flights of stairs, and returned to full day office work. After three months, a repeat MRI showed significant improvement (Figure 32). Mr D continues his physiotherapy stretches and maintenance sessions of USGDN once in 4 to 6 weeks. He leads an active personal and professional life, goes for family holidays, thus fulfilling all the health-related quality of life (HRQOL) criteria, which include the daily necessities of personal life, professional life, social life, recreational activities, sports and more.

Reversal of Structural changes of the spine with botox and USGDN

Patient after a back surgery: A patient with persistent back pain after disc surgery had to walk extensively in hilly terrain for his home visits as a doctor and was considering early retirement, since treatments in various pain clinics had failed to provide relief. After detailed history, examination, and discussion, he agreed for a thermal RF of the nerves that supply the facet, followed by USGDN to address the back muscles causing this pain. He was not really hopeful since three RFA procedures tried elsewhere had not helped. He was pleasantly surprised that he felt better after RFA this time and as the USGDN sessions proceeded he felt much better in about a month and was able to resume his job in Oman and lead a normal lifestyle. RFA+USGDN was repeated after three years. Five years later when he came for a visit, he asserted confidently that he no longer required any treatment but had, in fact, was able to undertake a fairly strenuous trek. Thereafter, he brought his mother for treatment of an old-age-related spinal canal narrowing called lumbar canal stenosis. Epidural steroid injection reduced the pressure on her spinal nerves and botox injection reduced the muscle pains caused by the nerve compression.

In 2022, the patient had a recurrence of back pain after 11 years. The MRI showed a mild disc prolapse and spondylolisthesis where his vertebrae had slipped forward in two places. Epidural steroid, botox, and USGDN to alter the tensioning of muscles at the front and back of the spine to allow his vertebrae to go back to their place, were suggested. After seeing how his mother benefited from botox, he was only too happy to receive botox. Within a month he was totally comfortable and resumed an active lifestyle. Three months later, the ultrasound of back muscles showed significant improvement. A repeat X-ray after six months was better and he was quite happy with the clinical improvement. He works out every day (a judicious mix of aerobics, gym, and yoga), does a full day's work, regularly goes for holidays, goes trekking without any pains or limitations thus fulfilling the five-fold criteria in the HRQOL.

Botox and USGDN for cancer pain

The neuromyopathic pains of cancer benefit remarkably from botox injections. Experiences with two following patients exemplify the benefits of viewing cancer pains with the perspective of neuromyopathy. The same mechanism of pain referral operates for two disparate structures in different organs, the liver and abdomen, and the meningeal coverings of the brain, to the final common expressor of pain, the muscle.

Botox and USGDN for liver cancer

FP, a doctor friend sought answers for a Catch-22 situation for her brother who needed morphine neuromodulators and fentanyl patches to make his post-surgical and chemotherapy stage-4 liver cancer pains bearable, but the opioids were slowing his gut movements to cause a known but rare complication of intestinal obstruction. This surgical emergency required frequent hospital admissions, morphine cessation, intravenous hydration and gut decompression with a nasogastric tube. FP urgently sought some alternative to this *impasse*. It was explained to her that pains from the abdominal organs were expressing themselves as spasms in the back and abdominal muscles. Ultrasound guided botox into all the muscles that form the abdominal oval, including muscles of the back, the six packs, and the oblique muscles would relieve his pain. After two days, when his intestinal obstruction had cleared, the botox injection was administered. The first few sessions of USGDN addressed several painful MTrPs in the back and the intercostal muscles between the ribs overlying the liver. Gradually, the pains decreased to such an extent that he could go off the fentanyl patches. He was very happy to resume his work to put his affairs in order. He was doing very well but unfortunately 6 months later, he succumbed to covid.

Botox for metastasized brain cancer

A neurosurgeon referred SR, for pain relief from a lymphoma that had spread to his brain. SR was a strapping young handsome and tall man with a clean shaven head and a body that was beginning to emaciate, as a prelude to a fast-approaching end from cancer. He complained of severe pain in the neck and head despite the neuromodulator medications and opioids. In fact, he was on high doses of medications and was drowsy, appearing confused, but spoke very coherently when discussing his treatment options. It was explained to him that although the brain is the final receptacle for all bodily sensations, it has no sensation in itself, and the brain metastases was unlikely to cause pain. However, the pains that he was experiencing could be because the metastases were directly involving the meninges or stretching them. The meninges are very sensitive because of the rich supply of nerves and meningeal irritation can cause headaches by referring their pain to the muscles of the head and neck. Based on this surmise, botox injection into the neck and scalp muscles under ultrasound vision would be given and followed up with USGDN to address any stragglers. He grasped the concept of pain referral from the meninges to the muscles and wanted to proceed immediately. Two days later, he was jubilant. He had no pain and had reduced the opioids, so his head felt a lot lighter, and he had resumed writing his memoirs! His only question was, did he really need the needling? It was reiterated that there would be some muscle fibres with MTrPs, which would have escaped the botox effect and if they were not relaxed by the USGDN, his pains could return. He did have some painful muscles, while most other areas were completely painless to needle entry, so the explanation was vindicated. He was very appreciative of the pain relief, and one day he asked, "Doc, now that my pain is gone, I feel that my cancer must be gone too, should I do a repeat MRI to check?" He was advised to wait another month as it was only two months since his last MRI. Another time he shared his thoughts, "Doc, I was told that my pain was untreatable because there were no interventions for it. I had resigned to suffering that terrible agony for whatever little life I had left. But here I am, pain-free after the botox injection and USGDN! Your different perspective of muscles being the paramount pain generators should become the norm so that patients like me, all over the world, can benefit. Would you be willing to do a podcast with my friend who does podcasts with a pan-global audience"? But alas, SR had an episode of aspiration pneumonia 4 days later and was no more after a fortnight.

References

[1] Devriese, P. 1999. On the discovery of *Clostridium botulinum*. J. Hist. Neurosci. 8: 43–50. doi: 10.1076/jhin.8.1.43.1774.

[2] Drachman, D.B. 1965. Pharmacological denervation of skeletal muscle in chick embryos treated with botulinum toxin. Trans Am. Neurol. Assoc. 90: 241–242.

[3] Jabbari, B. 2016. History of botulinum toxin treatment in movement disorders. Tremor and Other Hyperkinetic Movements 6. doi: 10.7916/D81836S1.

[4] Nigam, P.K. and A. Nigam. 2010. Botulinum toxin. Indian J. Dermatol. 55: 8–14.

[5] França, K., A. Kumar, M. Fioranelli et al. 2017. The history of Botulinum toxin: from poison to beauty. Wiener Medizinische Wochenschrift 167(1): 46–48.

[6] Erbguth, FJ. 2008. From poison to remedy: the chequered history of botulinum toxin. Journal of Neural Transmission 115(4): 559–565.

[7] Bach, K. and R. Simman. 2022. The Multispecialty toxin: a literature review of Botulinum toxin. Plastic and Reconstructive Surgery Global Open 10(4).

Chapter 5

Intuitive Learning of Complex Regional Pain Syndrome (CRPS)

Complex Regional Pain Syndrome (CRPS), has remained a major enigma amongst specialists on pain management. This chapter provides a gist of the publications on CRPS;[1-11] from 2003 to 2023, on lessons learnt from the patients, the intricacies of the disease, its symptoms, and what treatments work.

The IASP defines CRPS Type 1 as, "A variety of painful conditions following injury, which appear in a region and have a distal predominance of abnormal findings, exceeding in both magnitude and duration; the expected clinical course of the inciting event, often results in significant impairment of motor functions and showing variable progressions over time." It may involve any part of the body but is more common in the limbs, which look swollen, angry, red, and is usually extremely painful as if there is some infection and inflammation[12] (Figure 33). However, blood investigations suggestive of infection are negative.

CRPS exhibits neuropathic features like shocks, tingling, insect-crawling sensation, pulling pain, numbness, and paradoxical pain in a 'numb' area. The skin becomes dark, tender, and oversensitive; even a light touch or a breeze is painful. The most striking symptom, however, is severe stiffness associated with weakness; patients cannot bend the fingers, touch the thumb to fingertips to pick up objects, make a fist to grasp objects, or perform fine hand functions, like writing. Patients

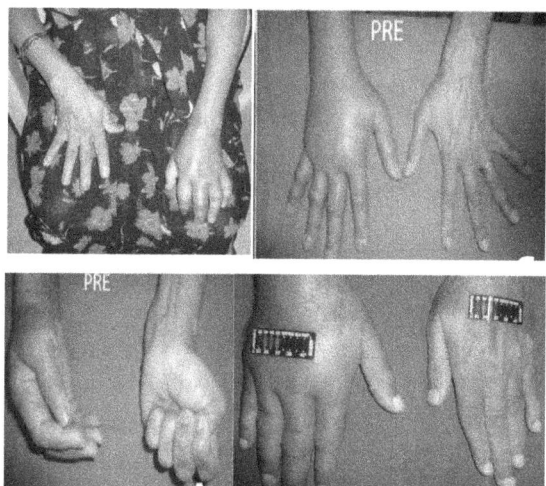

Figure 33. The swollen, stiff, dark, and warm CRPS hand in three different patients.

avoid the slightest movement due to extreme pain. Limiting movement reduces the pain and swelling but increases stiffness. The moment the patient tries to move the affected part, the swelling and pain returns with renewed vigour. In lower-limb CRPS, weight-bearing becomes extremely painful with highly restricted foot and ankle movements, which prevents standing and walking.

CRPS is a perplexing conglomeration of signs and symptoms with an uncertain cause. How or why the disease develops and how to treat it successfully, remains unknown. Currently, the diagnosis is based on clinical symptoms (what the patient reports) and signs (what the physician verifies during examination) laid down by IASP called the clinical diagnostic criteria (CDC) or Budapest criteria. CRPS diagnosis remains problematic because not all signs or symptoms may manifest at the time of examination.[13] No investigation consistently confirms diagnosis or prognosis. Muscle MRI as an investigation has been discarded as inconsistent, too expensive, and unavailable at the bedside. X-rays show bone loss (osteopenia and osteoporosis) only in late-stage CRPS. Three-phase bone scan findings of higher radioactive material uptake in the third phase may be inconsistent among patients. We have reported the efficacy of MSKUSG as a diagnostic investigation in 2013[9] but other researchers are yet to explore this possibility.

CRPS outcomes are bleak because interventional treatments are either quasi-effective or ineffective but are continued in select patients because nothing else is available. One such treatment is the implantation of a spinal cord stimulator (SCS), an expensive device with attendant maintenance requirements and complications. SCS replaces the pain with paraesthesia (tingling sensation) but does not address the weakness, stiffness, or the ensuing CRPS disability. Opioids are routinely prescribed to make life easier for the patients, but unfortunately neuropathic pains are refractory to opioids and this may lead to dose escalation and addiction. Historically, physiotherapy has been quasi-effective but the progress plateaus over time. Some patients find it too painful and feel that it worsens their symptoms and discontinue it.

Different approach to CRPS

Our approach to CRPS has been strikingly different. All our 220 patients till date, have experienced relief from all the symptoms, which is very significant given the nature of the uncommon problem. The patients not only got relief from pain, but they also experienced reversal of the disability, which was hitherto unheard of in CRPS literature.

Face-to-face with CRPS

The experience with CRPS started in early 2004. Two elderly patients presented with CRPS with severe pain and disability, were totally unresponsive to medication. Both patients were down-to-earth, self-effacing people who had seen life and were not ones to exaggerate their suffering. Yet they reported excruciating pain and crippling hand stiffness. At that time, CRPS was a complete enigma. The vast literature including textbooks on pain, was less than helpful, highly confusing, with unproven hypotheses about the cause, and how and why CRPS manifests as it does. Unfortunately, recommended treatments based on these hypotheses, such as medication and sympathetic ganglion block (SGB) had inconsistent efficacy. Most systemic reviews concluded that the exact mechanism of the Stellate ganglion block (SGB) action was uncertain and who would benefit was unpredictable. If SGB worked, the pain was considered to be sympathetically maintained (SMP), and treatment was repeated as needed. When SGB did not work, the pain was called sympathetically independent (SIP) and SGB played no further role.

It would be wrong to simply assume that these two patients had SMP, which an SGB would relieve. Even if SGB was effective, sooner

Table Effectiveness of USGDN in 220 patients of Complex regional pain syndrome (CRPS).

Anatomical location	Patient No, CRPS type	Budapest criteria	
Upper extremity (UE)	168 patients 50 men 118 women 160 CRPS-1 patients and 8 CRPS-2 patients	+ve in all 168	Budapest criteria, treatment given, disability of arm, shoulder and hand score (DASH), lower extremity function score (LEFS), ultrasound changes and post treatment Budapest criteria return to prior lifestyle. The first 8 patients received only stellate (sympathetic ganglion) block (SGB) and continuous brachial plexus block (CBPB) and no USGDN. All 8 required 8-10weeks of CBPB which was difficult to maintain. 1 patient failed to improve. Later 23 patients received SGB, CBPB and USGDN. Addition of USGDN reduced the recovery time from 8-10 weeks to 3–6 weeks. Once the mechanism of co-contraction was understood we used USGDN as the sole treatment modality in the later 137 patients. We discontinued the blocks since all the complications were associated with the catheter used for CBPB and none with USGDN.
Post stroke CRPS	5 - All had upper extremity CRPS	+ve in all 5	Budapest criteria: Resolution of all the symptoms and signs that form Budapest criteria like sensory, sudomotor, vasomotor and motor manifestations were documented in 167 patients.
Bilateral CRPS	5 Upper extremity CRPS	+ve	Ultrasound demonstrated loss of outline, hyperechogenecity, reduction of muscle bulk in all patients. 7 patients with early CRPS with florid manifestations showed occasional muscle oedema and intermuscular effusions in patients. In some patients, the muscle disruption was limited to few muscles while patients with later CRPS showed marked changes in all the muscles. After 1 month of USGDN, all these muscles showed improvement with disappearance
Recurrent CRPS	2 Upper extremity CRPS	+ve	of muscle edema, intermuscular effusions, return of islands of hypoechoic muscle amidst hyperechoic fibrous tissue, returning definition of muscle outlines and increasing muscle bulk.
Paediatric age group	2 Upper extremity CRPS	+ve	All patients showed >80% improvement in DASH scores, range of motion with restoration of normal hand functions. >98% patients returned to prior lifestyle.

Table contd. ...

...Table contd.

Lower extremity (LE)	48 patients 20 men 28 women 1 teenager. 44 CRPS-1 patients and 4 CRPS-2 patients	+ve in all 48	In 38 patients continuous sciatic block was used along with USGDN. 10 patients received only USGDN. Lower extremity CRPS patients seemed to improve faster with continuous sciatic block which appeared to expedite and facilitate painless weight bearing. The ultrasound changes with CRPS were similar to upper extremity CRPS and their response to USGDN identical. Disability was assessed with lower extremity function score(LEFS). All patients showed resolution of all the symptoms and signs that form Budapest criteria like sensory, sudomotor, vasomotor and motor manifestations. > 80% improvement in LEFS with resumption of normal unaided walk in all the patients. > 98% patients returned to prior lifestyle.
Chest wall	4 men CRPS 1	+ve in 4	All the 4 patients showed resolution of all the sensory, sudomotor, vasomotor and motor symptoms and signs that form Budapest criteria with USGDN.

The pathology of CRPS appears to be primarily motor; with formation of abundant MTrPs and taut bands in the agonist/antagonist muscles such as flexor/extensors, supinator /pronators and adductor/abductors. The taut bands in these muscle groups impair reciprocal inhibition essential for smooth movements. The tautness in coworking muscles culminates in an abnormal co-contraction which severely impedes all extremity and digital movements. Attempted movements of muscles tethered by constant co-contraction leads to friction at the digital tenosynovial sheaths giving rise to inflammation. Thus, the motor impairment due to co-contraction forms the primary pathology of CRPS giving rise to tenosynovial inflammation. Budapest criteria are, but manifestations of tenosynovial inflammation presenting with all its classical features; namely rubor (redness, the vasomotor feature of CRPS), dolor (pain and other sensory features), calor (temperature asymmetry, another vasomotor feature) and tumor (swelling or sudomotor manifestation of CRPS).
Relaxation of the co-contracted agonist/antagonist muscles of the CRPS-affected limb by USGDN automatically reduces the tenosynovial friction and resolves the inflammatory tendinosis in the hand, thereby reversing the pain, sensory features, warmth, and swelling (vasomotor & sudomotor) AND allows a return of the normal coordination between the flexor (agonist) and extensor (antagonist) muscles with dramatic improvement of stiffness, weakness, and disability. Ultrasound documentation of structural disruption in CRPS-affected muscles as well as their reversal after USGDN supports this theory. [12-17]

DASH - Disability of arm shoulder hand score. LEFS-Lower extremity function score . MTrPs-myofascial trigger points .
Vas, L.C. 2022. Ultrasound guided dry needling: Relevance in chronic pain. J. Postgrad. Med. Jan 1; 68(1): 1.

or later, that effect would wear off. The patients could not be indefinitely dependent on temporarily effective interventions. To understand the complexity of sympathetic pain, it must be understood that the face, hands, and feet have the maximum density of nerves. This makes the face mobile, hands dexterous, and feet nimble, and as also the most sensitive parts of the body. Besides the sensory and motor nerves under voluntary control, there are sympathetic and parasympathetic nerves of the autonomic or involuntary nervous system, which cannot be controlled at will. In situations of extreme fear or danger, the sympathetic nerves divert blood supply from the skin (resulting in cold clammy hands) to muscles and increases the heart rate, to execute a fright-flight-fight response. Since danger and pain go hand in hand on many occasions, involvement of sympathetic nervous system in pains is routine (SMP). Empathy and sympathy are not only in human minds and thoughts, but nature has built them into the very body as a fundamental law of existence so that all parts of the body exist in complete harmony with each other. The sympathetic ganglion, which controls pains in the head, face, neck, and upper limb is the stellate ganglion (Figure 18) located in the front of the neck next to the trachea (windpipe) and oesophagus (food pipe). The sympathetic ganglion for the abdomen is the celiac ganglion located between the stomach and liver, and lumbar sympathetic ganglion for the lower limbs is located beside the lumbar vertebral body.

Along with the SGB, a continuous brachial plexus block (CBPB) could provide continuous pain relief to overcome the typical tendency of CRPS patients to avoid movement and permit effective physiotherapy. Continuous and complete pain suppression would also prevent recurrence by unwinding the spinal sensitization. Placing and maintaining peripheral nerve catheters for continued pain relief and tunnelling the catheter away under the skin so that the needle entry site is covered by skin regrowth to minimize the infection risk[14] had been a part of routine pediatric anaesthesia practice at Wadia children's hospital. The CBPB catheter had to be tunnelled since it was imperative to ensure certain and lasting pain relief of the entire limb.

After a detailed discussion of CBPB risks and benefits, both patients wanted to go ahead. SGB achieved about 30 per cent pain relief, but CBPB resulted in instantaneous and dramatic relief from pain and distress. The initial bolus dose of lignocaine (a short-acting local anaesthetic) was followed by 2 ml/hour of a low concentration of a long-acting local anaesthetic bupivacaine from an elastomeric pump.

Both patients started eating and sleeping normally, and regained interest in life. But perplexingly, the stiffness, the limitation of hand movement persisted even after the limb was totally pain-free, making it obvious that in CRPS, *the pain and muscle stiffness were distinct entities.* This was a revelation because most literature on CRPS intuitively implies that patients avoid movement because of pain. But CBPB clearly uncoupled the connection and indicated that the stiffness that was restricting movements was independent of the pain.

After a week, the stiffness still impeded the range of movements (ROM), as if the patients were relearning how to move the clumsy limb. Both the physiotherapist and the patients had to work very hard for every millimetre of movement. Both the patients required anaesthesia with extra 12–15 ml of 2 per cent lignocaine to allow the physiotherapist to passively mobilize the finger joints beyond what the patients could do voluntarily.

The plan was to remove the catheters after one week because the longer a foreign body is retained inside the body, the higher is the risk of infection. Both patients were most reluctant to let go of the CBPB, which had made them so comfortable. They were ready to accept the potential risk of infection. Finally, the lady's catheter was removed uneventfully at 45 days (Figure 34) and the man's at 60 days since he had much more stiffness and pain. Their perseverance had increased the movements of the wrist, metacarpophalangeal joints (MCPJ, the proximal knuckles), and interphalangeal joints (IPJ, the two distal knuckles) of the fingers to make a fist, an ability essential for practically every hand function. Both recovered complete use of the hand for all the necessary daily activities (Figure 35).

After these two patients were successfully treated, it was obvious that something important had been achieved because it is unusual for CRPS and the associated disability to be completely cured, almost as if the patients never had any problems. The following year four more patients benefited with the same treatment. The recurrent issue in all these patients was the movement difficulty, which took six-to-eight weeks to resolve even after being completely pain-free with CBPB. The physiotherapist could not bend the fingers passively into a fist. With excessive pressure the patients would suffer total CRPS recurrence with an angry, swollen red hand. After a day or two's rest, the symptoms would subside allowing the resumption of physiotherapy. Thus, physiotherapy was like a double-edged sword causing a yo-yo of symptoms. The

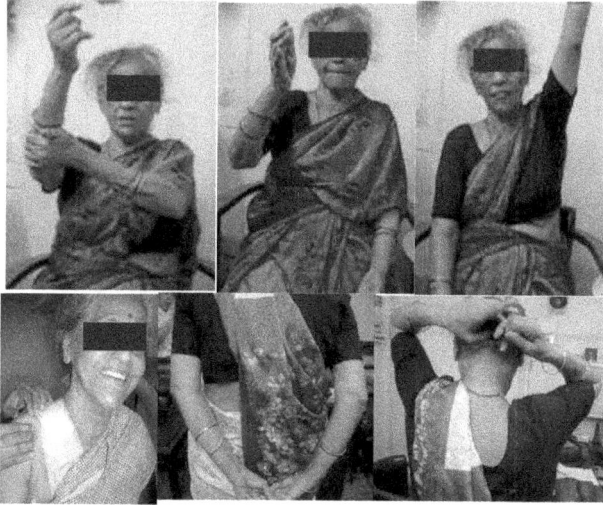

Figure 34. Top row: Painful and stiff right shoulder-hand syndrome. The right image shows the normal movement at left shoulder. Bottom row left: Pain-free patient smiling after the stellate ganglion and continuous brachial plexus block.Middle and right: After 45 days, patient is pain-free, without disability.

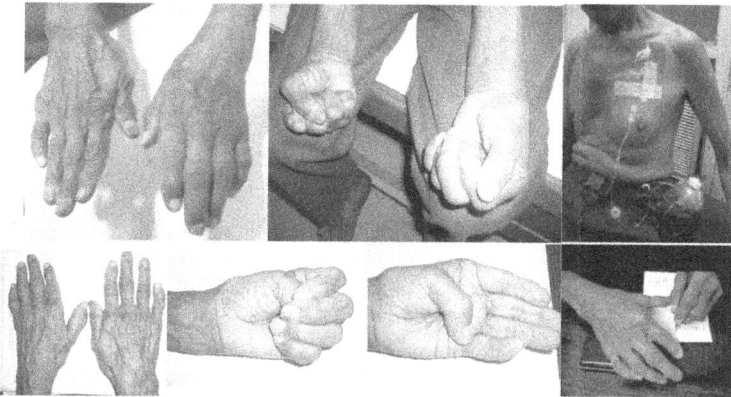

Figure 35. Top row: Swollen, painful, stiff left hand. The right image shows the catheter connected to an elastomeric pump. Bottom row: Sixty pain-free days enabling physiotherapy, made activities possible.

saving grace was the CBPB, which kept the patients pain-free despite the swelling. Physiotherapists found it intriguing to work with CRPS patients rendered pain-free by CBPB. Over time, the physiotherapist and patients understood that a 3–4^0 ROM increase per session was the limit

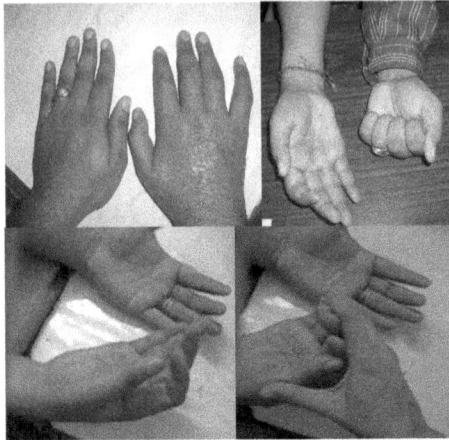

Figure 36. Top row: Cold, stiff, useless and (hence painless) right hand after two years of CRPS. Bottom row: Unable to move fingers after one month of continuous analgesia.

of pushing the hand. Once the physiotherapist achieved a better ROM of passive movement, the patients could follow through with active movements within the pain-free ROM. This was a slow and painstaking process, but they were motivated by the comfort provided by CBPB.

Each patient re-affirmed the conviction that the more crucial problem of CRPS was stiffness and not pain. Once a patient regained hand function, the CBPB could be discontinued without the pain recurring. The movement difficulty had to be because something was intrinsically wrong with the CRPS muscle. Blocking the nerves was an indirect, roundabout way of addressing the stiff muscle, but it was continued because there was no clue about how the stiffness could be cured. At least, CBPB made the patient completely pain-free and physiotherapy could reduce the stiffness and restore the hand function.

In 2005, the seventh patient, a young shopkeeper suffering from CRPS for two years, did not respond to the treatment, even after a month of CBPB. Physiotherapy had no impact on his severely stiff but painless cold right hand fixed in extension (Figure 36). The treatment ended after an accidental catheter extrusion.

The muscle pathology

The intrinsic muscle pathology was becoming a nemesis as the key problem in CRPS. USGDN was already being used in various pain conditions with significant success but not in CRPS because of the influence of the extensive (but unhelpful) literature on CRPS, stating that it was a nervous disease. But the seventh patient brought home the point that muscles had to be proactively addressed.

Successful out-of-the-box hypothesis and treatment

The opportunity to test the hypothesis of an intrinsic muscle involvement in CRPS arrived with the next patient in 2006, with spontaneous shoulder-hand syndrome. SGB and CBPB relieved the pain, the swelling (Figure 37), and sleep disturbances. She was very happy with the improvement but rather miffed at the insistence to continue treatment to regain all movements. She was unable to lift her arm because of a 'catch', as she described it, in the armpit, overlying the coracobrachialis, pectoralis minor, and the biceps. The USGDN needles were placed in these muscles to see if that made any difference to the pain and movements. After the needles were removed, the patient raised her hand all the way up without pain! (Figure 38). The results of continued USGDN of the neck and upper limb for the following week were nothing short of miraculous. She was completely cured in just 18 days (Figure 38) while the first six patients had taken 45–60 days and the seventh had failed to recover! It was uncertain whether this was a fluke or a lucky hunch. Well, there was only one way of finding out! In the

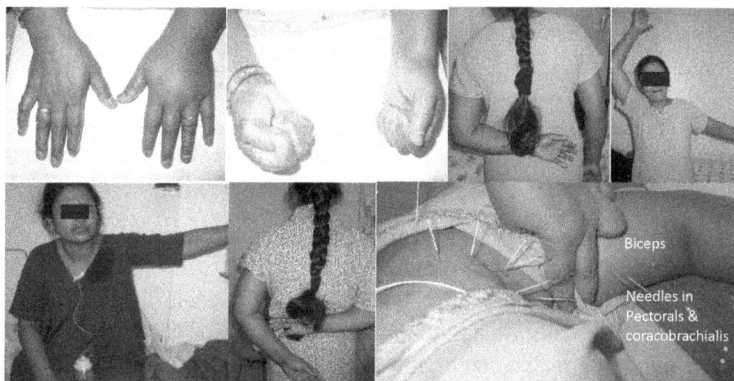

Figure 37. Top row: Spontaneous shoulder-hand syndrome with a swollen painful useless left upper limb. Bottom row: The 2 left images show persistent limitation at left shoulder. The right image shows dry needling of biceps, coracobrachialis, and pectoral muscles.

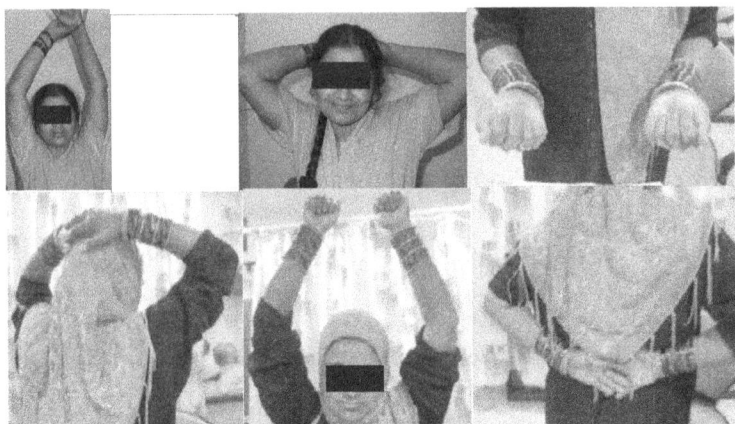

Figure 38. Top row: Instantaneous pain relief by USGDN restored shoulder movements. Bottom row: CRPS reversal at 18 days restored movement, relieved pain, and swelling.

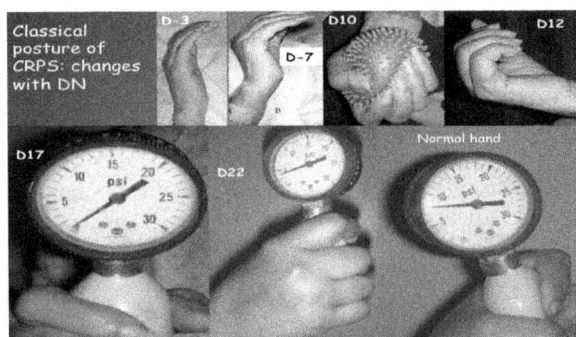

Figure 39. Top row: Serial images of CRPS recovery from complete disability to normalcy. Bottom On day 17 the grip strength is 0. but on day 22, the grip strength is 4 PSI, (pounds per square inch) sufficient for all daily activities by 22 days.

next few years, USGDN kept producing good results with clockwork precision in all the patients (Figure 39).

The motor recovery after USGDN brought home the realization of just how difficult the day-to-day activities are, for CRPS patients. It was a humbling realization of how one remains unaware of the dexterity and skill needed to perform the simplest activities like dressing, eating and writing. These simple, nearly involuntary actions that are taken for granted, become difficult or even impossible for CRPS patients. It was very sobering to watch the child-like thrill and excitement of the patients when they could suddenly perform the simplest acts like buttoning up shirts, fastening trousers or adjusting their clothes and hair, actions that are ridiculously easy for a healthy person.

The hows and whys of success

The dramatic efficacy of DN was great but we still had no idea why or how. No amount of mulling over this produced any answers and not wanting to look a gift horse in the mouth, USGDN was continued till the tenth patient, inadvertently provided the answers in 2007.

He was scheduled for surgery for cut tendons at the wrist after knife injuries. Fortunately, he consulted a senior doctor, an experienced and discerning hand surgeon, who diagnosed CRPS and referred him to us. Sonography confirmed that his tendons were intact. The CRPS was obvious on examination (Figure 40) with severely restricted movements but interestingly, on attempting to touch his thumb to the fingertips, he developed dystonia (coarse fluttering) of the fingers.

Observing this dystonia brought on a sudden thought, that this was actually the movement of the co-contracted muscles struggling against each other! This was an intuitive and instantaneous thought, not a logically reasoned-out conclusion. The term 'co-contraction' is not exactly a part of pain physician vocabulary although most would have studied it in

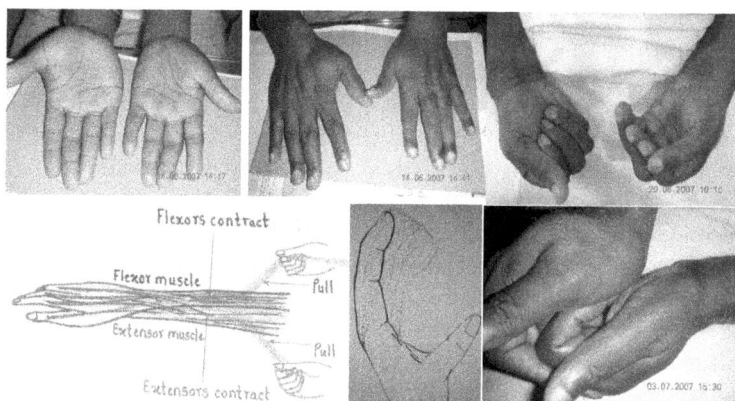

Figure 40. Top row: Narrow left CRPS hand with scar on the palm, colour asymmetry, swelling. Bottom left: Representation of flexor/extensor co-contraction causing CRPS stiffness. Middle: Severe dystonia of the fingers. Right: Gentle pressure on the fingers achieves full flexion.

physiology decades earlier. We had to look up the exact definition and explanation. Every movement requires work from two sets of muscles: one that causes the movement (the agonist) and another that opposes it (the antagonist). For example, bending the fingers by the finger flexors (agonist), requires relaxation of the finger extensors (antagonist). In co-contraction, both flexors and extensors contract simultaneously and forcefully. This aberration of two muscles with opposing functions contracting simultaneously was difficult to fathom and mulling over it did not provide any clarity till an explanation for this phenomenon was provided by Vasu my husband, a mechanical engineer. He immediately explained, "The flexor muscle, which is contracting, has to be *guided* by the extensor with an opposing function." But the question was, "Why can't the muscle do its work by itself, why does it need an opponent for doing its work?" Then he explained the principle of 'guiding' as it is called in mechanical parlance, "Any movement, unless there is guidance by an opposite force, will be erratic and jerky, and uncontrolled. The opposing force holds it back (rein it in as it were), with just that little bit of resistance, so that there is a smooth control to the movement, which happens just as we want it." For the smooth movement of the finger, when the flexor contracts to bend the finger, the extensor should relax just enough to make the movement of the flexor muscle smooth and balanced. It took a while to assimilate this concept in its entirety, but once understood, it was awe inspiring, the way Nature has developed such sophisticated and intricate controls for the mind-boggling, countless movements of the body, with such finesse and 24×7 precision, to be "just so". Every movement in the body has pairs of agonists and antagonists (flexor/extensor, pronator/supinator, adductor/abductor) controlled by a physiological process called reciprocal inhibition for exquisitely controlled and streamlined movements. The simple elegance of this concept is absolutely reflective of the perfection and simplicity of Nature, and it became intuitively obvious that with these thoughts one was finally on the right track.

Physiological co-contraction is a voluntary action that is held, maintained, and terminated at will. It is painless and sustained easily, to provide a stable base to allow the performance of some complex movements. For example, the wrist has to be fixed in a slightly extended position to form a stable base so that the fingers holding a pen can flex and extend repetitively at the interphalangeal joints (IPJ), to perform the delicate, rapid movements of writing (Figure 41).

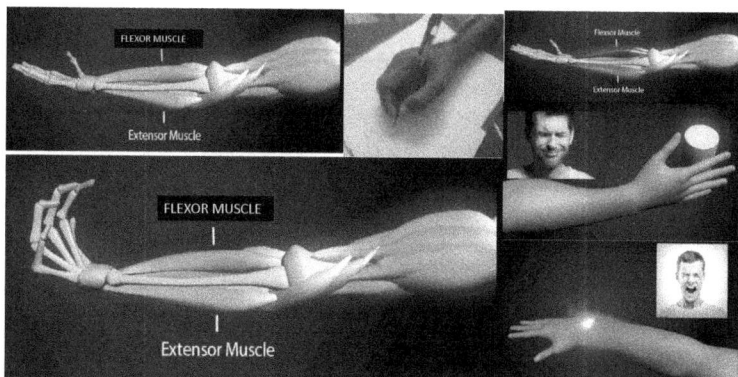

Figure 41. Top left: Flexors and extensors relaxed in neutral position. Middle: Wrist fixed in slight extension by a physiological flexors/extensor co-contraction allows the fingers to write. Bottom left: When the flexors contract, the extensors relax to allow finger flexion. Right: Intense, severely painful co-contraction in CRPS precludes patient from grasping a glass. Inordinate effort at hand flexion causes frictional inflammation of extensor tendon sheaths to produce swelling, warmth, and pain of CRPS.

The intriguing concept of constant co-contraction as a working hypothesis for CRPS implies a very different category of abnormality, which induces a contradictory combination of weakness associated with stiffness (Figure 41). It is,

- highly exaggerated
- extremely painful
- constantly present
- uncontrollable—the patient has no control whatsoever on it.

Any attempt to overcome this co-contraction and perform a purposeful movement exaggerates it in the form of dystonic movements.

The concept of co-contraction explained why CRPS patients struggle so much with any movement. It also explained the dramatic success of USGDN, which relaxes all the muscles in a graded and systematic manner, actually reduces the co-contraction, restores reciprocal inhibition to replace co-contraction with the delicate coordination required for normal movements.

USGDN under the cover of CBPB relieved the abnormal co-contraction resulting in complete reversal of dystonia within a week, sensory and other problems in a month, and the patient returned home, to Nigeria, with a normal hand.

But it was still uncertain as to how or why co-contraction was connected to the inflamed-looking CRPS hand, which is responsible for producing the clinical diagnostic criteria of IASP. As more and more patients with dystonia, pain, and all the CRPS manifestations were seen between 2006 and 2009, more pieces of the CRPS jigsaw fell into place. The logic of co-contraction and DN was obvious to us after witnessing the daily success of DN relieving CRPS, but the expert reviewers, scrutinizing the papers on the efficacy of USGDN in CRPS submitted for publication, rejected them outright. Most of them had probably never held a filiform needle in their hands. Entrenched in the prevailing worldview of CRPS, they could not accept these revolutionary, out-of-box views although the pre- and post-treatment pictures told their own story (Figures 34, 35 and 37–40). There was not much that could be done without some objective evidence that could prove the co-contraction hypothesis.

Tangible proof with objective demonstration

In 2009, when an ultrasonography (USG) machine was brought for demonstration, it provided the opportunity to see if musculoskeletal ultrasonography could objectively demonstrate the muscle issues of CRPS. There were two CRPS patients at the clinic that day and what the sonography showed was mind blowing! The USG unequivocally showed, in black and white, what had been suspected, believed, and written about, that there was a discernible and intrinsic muscle abnormality in CRPS. A normal muscle shows clearly delineated outlines and generally appears black with bright streaks of the connective tissue framework that holds the muscle fibres in well-defined bundles. In stark contrast, the muscles after two years of CRPS appeared as a sheet of white (fibrotic) tissue, without any form or shape or discernible outlines. The muscle bulk was shrunken in the CRPS hand as compared to the normal hand (Figure 42).

Fifteen days of USGDN seemed to bring back black 'islands' of the muscle into the white fibrotic tissue in this and subsequent patients. Reappearance of the muscle coincided with normalization of movements in the stiff hand. This meant that USGDN was actually regenerating the muscle fibres within the fibrous mass (Figure 42). How and why these changes occurred in the muscle was still a mystery, but thereafter, it became a part of CRPS treatment protocol to routinely document the muscle changes in every patient before USGDN, at 15- and 30-day intervals, and after full recovery. Videos of the sequence

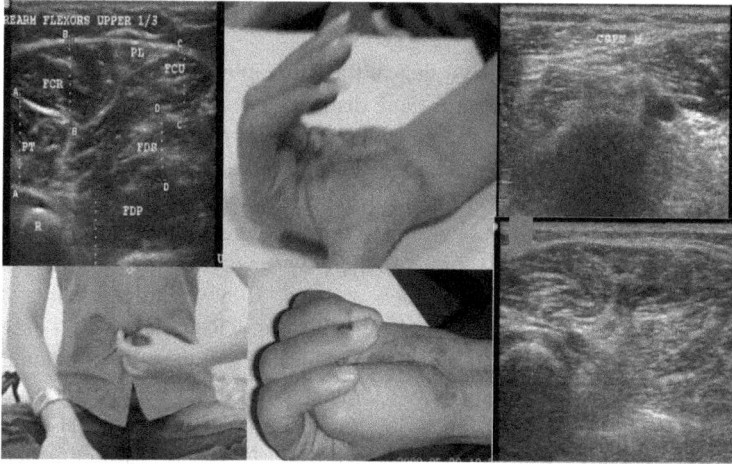

Figure 42. Top left: Hypoechoic (black) normal muscle with well-defined muscle outlines and hyperechoic (white) streaks of connective tissue. The lettering indicates individual muscles. Middle: Inability to make a fist. Right: Structurally disrupted CRPS muscles as white fibrous tissue. Bottom left: Normal functional hand. Middle: Fisting. Right: Return of black muscle bulk and clear outlines.

of sonographic events in the muscle at the introduction of the needle were also documented. The variety of clinical presentations were documented with still photos and videos, picturizing the limitations of movements, the grip strength (pressures generated on a dynamometer), and finger pressure with the pinch gauge. The ROM at all the joints of the limb was documented with a goniometer. The limb functionality was documented with the disability of the arm, shoulder, and hand (DASH) score. CRPS patients start out with a high DASH score (60–100) and as they improve, their scores come down to 10–20. This systematic documentation was crucial for the scientific community to verify and accept these findings to ensure that this effective treatment could be available to CRPS patients worldwide. This process of documentation is now part of the Ashirvad protocol.

Our first article, "Ultrasound appearance of CRPS muscles", was provisionally accepted in 2011, but was published in January 2013 in the journal, *Pain Practice*.[9] The reasons for this delay was the unusual nature of the topic, the potential of ultrasound as a diagnostic investigation in CRPS, which had no confirmatory investigation at the time. Reviewers raised several queries, which had to be satisfactorily answered; the saving grace was the 31 pictures, which irrefutably told their convincing story, in black and white.

Another problem was that ultrasonography of CRPS muscles straddled over two disparate and distinct specialties, pain medicine and ultrasonography. The reviewers were pain specialists who had no expertise in the diagnostic applications of ultrasound and the actual experts in ultrasonography had no experience with CRPS. Until the publication of these findings, there was no examination of muscles with ultrasound in CRPS. In 2009, there were very few pain specialists who used ultrasonography in their practice. They would certainly not be familiar with the structural changes seen in CRPS. This was a case of accidentally venturing into a highly specialized unexplored domain because CRPS work involved two diverse realms, CRPS and diagnostic USG. Even in 2023, ten years later, all the publications on this topic are exclusively from the Ashirvad group.[1-11] No other research group explored the USG changes in CRPS either to refute or corroborate the findings, although they have since been cited over 31 times by different authors. Addition of USG into the armamentarium of CRPS treatment opened the door to the hitherto unexplored world of muscle pathology in CRPS, which provided many answers to explain the enigma of CRPS "writer's cramp" and many other chronic pains.[15]

The connection between co-contraction and the inflamed-looking hand of CRPS: Inflammation is cited in CRPS literature as an important finding but never with reference to muscles. It has been attributed to neuroinflammation to explain the increased levels of inflammatory mediators demonstrated in the CSF and the venous blood of the CRPS limb as compared to the normal hand. Inflammation in the CSF is surmised to track down from the spinal cord to the peripheral nerves of the hand to express itself as the inflamed red swollen CRPS hand. However, the interventions that address this hypothetical neuroinflammation with anti-inflammatory steroids at SGB may not work at all (SIP) or may only work temporarily in SMP. Single-shot nerve blocks and even CBPB have no effect on motor problems. Both SGB and CBPB rely heavily, and sometimes unsuccessfully (as in the seventh patient), on physiotherapy to improve functionality and have to be sustained for 40 to 70 days for improving the highly restricted movements. The first seven patients with SGB and CBPB unequivocally demonstrated the dichotomy of pain and stiffness in CRPS with completely pain-free yet severely stiff hands. Only after USGDN was added to the SGB+CBPB combination, they showed dramatic improvement of CRPS. CBPB was used for 40 patients while the understanding of USGDN in relieving co-contraction was still being refined. Two patients had accidental catheter extrusions at days 5 and 10 but they went on to complete recovery because of USGDN. This data indicated that the effects of nerve blocks are confined to partial and/or temporary pain relief and play only a secondary role in addressing the CRPS symptoms and signs that form the Budapest diagnostic criteria of CRPS, particularly of the motor (movement impairment), sudomotor (swelling of hand accompanied with excessive sweating), and the vasomotor (redness and increased temperature). Thus, neuroinflammation does not comprehensively explain all the CRPS manifestations; it neither acknowledges nor attempts to explain the muscle stiffness.

Ashirvad understanding: CRPS patients have a very clear and specific description of their pain. They seldom complain of any significant forearm pain, where the co-contracted muscles are, but always point to their fingers and wrists as the primary painful areas.

How and why does a co-contracted forearm muscle produce swelling, warmth, and pain in the hand? And why exactly does relaxing the forearm muscles by USGDN relieve the symptoms of a CRPS hand? USG provided the answer—the hand swelling is due to fluid collection (effusion) around the tendons of the flexor/extensor muscles in the hand. There is no swelling under the skin, superficial to the tendons (Figure 43). The highly complex, flexor and extensor tendons of the fingers have the super smooth cover of a synovial sheath, with an extremely rich nerve supply. It responds to the overstretching and strain of moving the co-contracted muscles with local friction and inflammation called tenosynovitis. Repeated friction and overstretching with tenosynovitis releases inflammatory mediators, which increase the swelling around the tendons. Tenosynovitis reciprocally worsens the already present flexor/extensor co-contraction, which in turn worsens the tenosynovial strain with further inflammation, forming a vicious circle.

The limb affected by CRPS experiences trauma every time the patient attempts to use the hand or do physical therapy and the increased friction feeds into this vicious circle explaining the repeated exacerbation of symptoms. Patients have no CRPS symptoms as long as the hand is immobilized in a plaster cast. The problems of pain and swelling start only during the mobilization phase, after the cast is removed, when they try to move the hand.

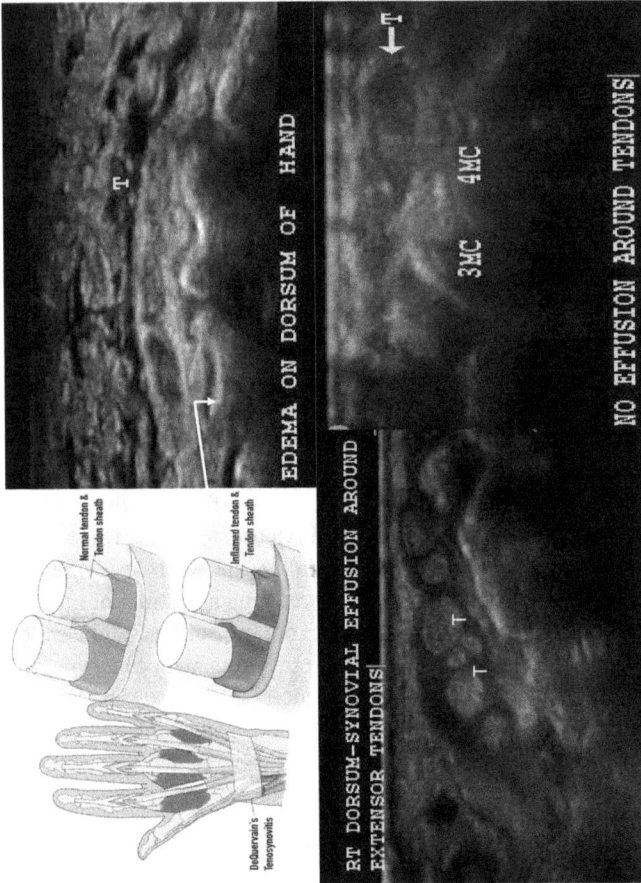

Figure 43. Top left: White extensor tendons covered by the grey synovial sheath. Right: Fluid collection beneath the skin but none around the tendons in a non-CRPS patient. Bottom left: Tenosynovitis causes black fluid collection around white tendons (T). Right: Disappearance of fluid after USGDN.

Co-contraction explains the puzzling off-and-on occurrence of the sudomotor and vasomotor features of CRPS as mentioned in the Budapest criteria. The explanation became evident when one of the patients, who had neither the sudomotor nor the vasomotor symptoms on her first visit, developed a red angry-looking hand of florid CRPS after the absolute pain relief from CBPB uncoupled the pain from the motor impairment. She passively forced the painless hand into a fist exacerbating tenosynovial friction and inflammation, which manifested as vasomotor and sudomotor symptoms of CRPS (Figures 42, 44), which responded to USGDN.

By relaxing the co-contracted muscles and restoring coordination, USGDN, reduces the tenosynovial friction or inflammation and actually makes physiotherapy a cakewalk. Any aggravation of the tenosynovitis caused by an intensive but productive session of physiotherapy, can be reversed with the next session of USGDN, which predictably relaxes the agonist and antagonist muscles to reduce the tenosynovitis. This predictability of pain relief empowers the patient to work confidently with the physiotherapist, making graded improvement an achievable goal.

The observations in CRPS and the patients' inputs were so absorbing that hours together would be spent with the early patients. Accepting their feedback on what worked for them and how, and what did not and why, and puzzling out the whys and hows with each patient added to the cumulative knowledge that demystified CRPS at Ashirvad.

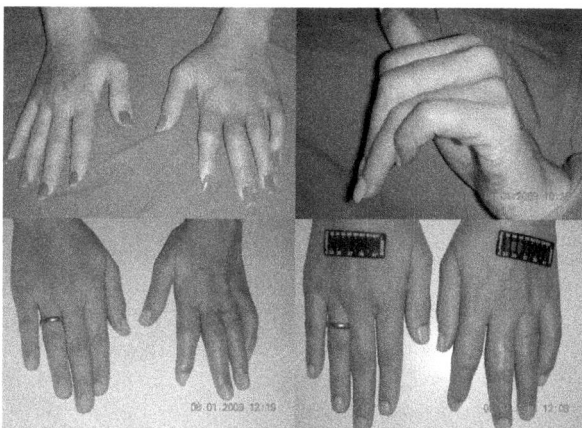

Figure 44. Top row: Painful, stiff, but uninflamed CRPS hand with restricted flexion. Bottom row: Aggressive physiotherapy triggered tenosynovitis (hot, shiny, swollen fingers).

The CRPS patients treated between 2004 and 2007 provided an unusual education of the vagaries of CRPS so that today, it can be routinely and confidently reversed with the certainty that the inflamed hand is a localized tenosynovitis consequent to the constant pull from the co-contracted forearm muscles and not some neuroinflammation from the spinal nerves, which mysteriously expresses itself in the hand.

Observations of USGDN in CRPS:

1) The earliest and most significant benefit is normalization of sleep because of substantial pain reduction within two-three USGDN sessions. Once relieved, the pain and stiffness do not recur with the original intensity even after intense physiotherapy.

2) The sensory symptoms such as hypersensitivity, allodynia (normal touch of clothes and breeze perceived as pain), insect-crawling, and shocks reduce within two to three USGDN sessions. Once relieved, these symptoms do not recur.

3) One of the most obvious and consistent findings in all CRPS patients is the reduction of skin temperature readings documented before and after an USGDN session. Any recurrence, after intensive physiotherapy, subsides after the next USGDN. After five to seven sessions, warmth does not recur.

4) The sudomotor symptom of swelling due to tenosynovial effusion in the hands disappears permanently after two weeks and six to seven USGDN sessions.

5) The colour changes take 10 to 15 days to normalize and do not recur.

6) The motor improvements sustain with each USGDN session, throughout the treatment period of 20 to 40 days. The dystonia is first replaced by purposeful movements. Since the entire limb and the neck muscles are addressed at every session, ROM improvements by a few degrees are seen at several joints after each session; wrist, MPJ and IPJs, elbow supination and extension, and all the shoulder movements to produce an overall improvement in the CRPS extremity.

Conclusion

The reason of USGDN's ability to specifically target the pathophysiology of CRPS became clear once it was understood that the Budapest criteria of CRPS were manifestations of tenosynovitis. The success with the 220 CRPS patients provided rare insights into this difficult problem with its seemingly bizarre and scientifically inexplicable presentations. Once the muscle pathology of co-contraction and its ramifications at the tendons and joints was acknowledged and understood, the entire gamut of CRPS presentations became easily explained. The seemingly inexplicable but consistent predictability of USGDN taught the intricacies of this condition in a very unusual way. The positive results were easy because they simply happened with USGDN, but the understanding of why these results came about was entirely another matter. Many manpower hours, days, and weeks were spent in futile perusals of literature to figure out probabilities and new theories to explain the process. A debt of immense gratitude is owed to the early patients who revealed the intricacies that were missing in the formidably vast literature on CRPS. Thanks to this insightful education, CRPS has become an easier problem to treat as compared to other pains.

References

[1] Vas, L. 2019. Commentary: Selective fiber degeneration of a patient with Complex Regional Pain Syndrome. Frontiers in Neuroscience 5(13): 19.

[2] Pai, R., L. Vas and M. Patnaik. 2018. Ultrasound guided intra-articular injection of radio-ulnar & radio-humeral joints; and dry needling of the affected limb muscles to relieve the fixed pronation deformity and secondary myofascial issues in a case of Complex Regional Pain Syndrome-type 1 (CRPS-1). Pain Practice 18(2): 273–282.

[3] Vas, L., R. Pai, D. Geete et al. 2018. Improvement in CRPS After deep dry needling suggests a role in myofascial pain. Pain Med. 19(1): 208–212.

[4] Vas, L.C., R. Pai and M. Pattnaik et al. 2016. Musculoskeletal ultrasonography in CRPS: Assessment of muscles before and after motor function recovery with dry needling as the sole treatment. Pain Physician 19(1): E163–179.

[5] Vas, L.C. and R. Pai. 2016. Musculoskeletal ultrasonography to distinguish muscle changes in complex regional pain syndrome type 1 from those of neuropathic pain: An observational study. Pain Practice 16(1): E1–E13.

[6] Vas, L. and R. Pai. 2016. Complex regional pain syndrome type 1 presenting as de Quervain's stenosing tenosynovitis. Pain Physician 19(1): E227–234.

[7] Vas, L. and R. Pai. 2014. Reversal of complex regional pain syndrome type 2 and the subsequent management of complex regional pain syndrome type 1 occurring after corrective surgery for residual ulnar claw. Pain Med. 15(6): 1059–1063.

[8] Vas, L. and R. Pai. 2012. Successful reversal of complex regional pain syndrome type 1 of both upper extremities in five patients. Pain Med. 13(9): 1253–1256.

[9] Vas, L.C., R. Pai and M. Radhakrishnan. 2013. Ultrasound appearance of forearm muscles in 18 patients with complex regional pain syndrome 1 of the upper extremity. Pain Practice. Jan; 13(1): 76–88.

[10] Vas, L. 2020. Retrospective review of successful and complete reversal of complex

regional pain syndrome and the associated disability of upper and lower extremities in 205 consecutive patients—Poster selected for oral presentation in the Amsterdam IASP conference in 2020. This was later presented virtually as a video and a poster due to Covid.

[11] Vas, L. 2007. Management of a Patient with CRPS-1 after total knee replacement. Indian Journal of Pain.

[12] Korwisi, B., A. Barke and R.D. Treede. 2021. Evidence-and consensus-based adaption of the IASP complex regional pain syndrome diagnostic criteria to the ICD-11 category of chronic primary pain: a successful cooperation of the IASP with the World Health Organization. Pain. Sep 1; 162(9): 2313–2314.

[13] Harden, R.N., S. Bruehl, R.S. Perez et al. 2010. Validation of proposed diagnostic criteria (the "Budapest Criteria") for complex regional pain syndrome. Pain. Aug 1; 150(2): 268–274.

[14] Vas, L. and V. Naik. 2000. Tunnelling of caudal Epidural catheters in infants. Paediatric Anaesthesia. 10: 149–154. This paper received the Danne Miller special citation and was chosen for publication in *Analgesia file*.

[15] Vas, L., R. Pai, N. Khandagale et al. 2015. Myofascial trigger points as a cause of abnormal cocontraction in writer's cramp. Pain Med. 16(10): 2041–2045.

Chapter 6
Physiotherapy, Yoga, and Pain

Physiotherapy is one of the pillars of pain management as are medication, interventional procedures, and counselling. When used with the correct methodology, along with yoga, it becomes indispensable in relieving pain.

Physiotherapy (PT)

PT is integral to pain management and comprises exercise, electrical modalities, and myofascial release protocols.

1. Exercises

The therapy starts with stretching exercises and graduates to strengthening exercises only after achieving good pain control with nerve blocks and USGDN. The exercises are kept simple with a judicious selection of simple stretches, which complement the effects of USGDN in reducing pain and stiffness so that the patients can do them correctly without precipitating cramps or muscle strain. Pain patients have serious muscle disturbances with a profusion of tender latent MTrPs, painful active MTrPs and taut bands, which are prone to injury. Normal healthy muscles are like new rubber bands with great elasticity but muscles with taut bands and MTrPs are like frayed, old rubber bands with minimal elasticity. Muscles are live structures with inbuilt protection against pain, which give a warning when contraction or stretching approaches harmful levels; this warning system helps to prevent major tears. But microtears occur routinely during several 'normal' activities, which overstretch the taut bands. Microtears are followed by inflammation with its hallmark features of rubor (redness), calor (warmth), dolour (pain), and tumour (swelling). Consequently, an already painful muscle becomes more painful and stiff when it is forcibly overstretched and even more so when overworked for strengthening, which in the worst-case scenario might even completely snap it. This is particularly relevant to elderly chronic pain patients, where even a small increase in activity to which they are unaccustomed, can produce a backlash of micro-injuries, inflammations, and pain recurrences, worsening the disability.

The patients are forewarned that nerve blocks relieve pain, making them feel that they can do anything, but blocks have no direct effect on the muscles, which are the main repository of pain and are far from normal. Patients have to be aware that unless they restrain themselves the pain will return with redoubled force. The general dictum is start low and go slow. The muscle stretches must stop the moment there is pain, that contrarily, has a slightly pleasant quality. If they go beyond the pleasant pain, they might develop microtears in the taut bands in the muscles and precipitate worse pain than before. They require at least four to six USGDN sessions before the muscles regain their elasticity to allow increased activity.

Simple stretches are gradually upgraded to complex exercises involving all the muscles that work together. Progressive resolution of the MTrPs enables patients to increase standing, walking, and daily activities. Only after pain is completely reduced, strengthening exercises are introduced to further alleviate the disability. If patients can resolve their pain with exercises, they need not spend the time, effort, and money for continuing treatments.

Interesting cases

Lumbar canal stenosis: Mrs A with age-related narrowing of vertebral canal compressing the spinal cord and nerves [lumbar canal stenosis (LCS)], had back and buttock pain of 8/10 on a numerical rating scale (NRS) (0—no pain; 10—severe unbearable pain) and 7–9/10 pain in the back of her thighs, calves, and feet on standing for one minute and walking for two minutes. After one epidural steroid injection and one USGDN session, she could stand for five minutes and walk for seven minutes without pain. Her mood and self-confidence took a happy upswing with an overall pain reduction of 50%. But when she returned again for USGDN, she was very downcast and said plaintively, "Doctor, your block failed! I have been careful as you had cautioned me but I just twisted back to pick up my specs and the pain restarted!" Reaching back for something is an involuntary activity one does routinely but it was enough to push this lady, who was teetering on the brink of muscle insufficiency, back into her pre-treatment pain levels.

Anxiety about the return of pain: The patient's first comment was "your block has failed!" when actually it was a recurrence of only a fraction of the original pains. Even a 10 per cent recurrence of pain, is misinterpreted as treatment failure, a harbinger of disaster, which has not really happened but is triggered by the fear of relapse. This is called catastrophizing, creating or anticipating a catastrophe when there is none. An overriding fear of pain and its recurrence makes this reaction fairly common among chronic pain patients who seem to forget their pre-therapy pain levels.

Exercises and attitude: The anxious patient felt somewhat reassured when told that the block effect, "does not go anywhere" and the new sprain would respond to exercises. She retorted that her pain increased with exercise. But when she did the exercises under guidance, 30 minutes later, she had a relieved but incredulous look on her face. With great exuberance but rather disbelievingly, she said, "The pain is gone! I can hardly believe it!" Actually, she had sprained her *quadratus lumborum* muscle, a very powerful muscle deep in the back that attaches the ribcage to the pelvis and refers the pains down to the buttocks and thighs. The sudden spasm (sprain) caused a seeming recurrence of her original pains. All it required was to stretch the muscle and the pain disappeared making her understand that simple exercises can actually relieve pain. This understanding that they can regain some control over pain and have a hand in their personal pain management empowers patients tremendously. This also makes patients acknowledge the susceptibility of their muscles to relapse into pain and the power of USGDN, in systematically reducing the vulnerability.

Forget about exercising: Once the patients complete USGDN sessions and are pain-free, they need to be regular with exercises to avoid pain recurrences. Unfortunately, self-discipline is rather uncommon and there are many who return after a few years to confess, shamefacedly, that after feeling fine with the last treatment the regime of exercising became increasingly rare. Others reasoned that they were cured so there was no need to bother with exercises. Exercises are the first thing to be jettisoned when they can't find time with their busy lifestyle, excessive travels, and so on.

In-tune and disciplined: Fortunately, there are many patients with good self-discipline and who exercise regularly. Some of them are so self-aware that they suddenly turn up after months or years even when they have no pain, because they feel something is not right, and therefore think it is better to take a 'preventive' USGDN session This is where USGDN is invaluable; it reveals some tight jumpy muscles with multiple LTRs which act as pain generators while their repeat MRI may be normal or be actually better (Figure 32, Chapter 4). Once treated, they are not seen again for years. One lady, who resumed an active lifestyle after being bedridden with lower-back pain for months used USGDN prophylactically. She would want a USGDN session whenever she had a hunch that something was not right, usually after an excessive workload. Once she came saying, "Doctor I danced a lot at a family wedding so I want USGDN before anything goes wrong." Sure enough, she had quite a few muscle issues, which were resolved with three to four USGDN sessions.

This said, a few patients insist that physiotherapy exercises worsen their pains. A retired vice-president of a prominent bank sought treatment for back pains, which had not responded to treatments by her orthopaedic surgeon son-in-law. She reported a consistent 80 per cent pain relief in response to two test doses of local anaesthetic to the nerves that supply the arthritic facet joints and also to radiofrequency ablation (RFA) of the same nerves. She was quite happy with the relief and with USGDN but not with physiotherapy which she felt brought on pain recurrences within four to five days after each USGDN session. She did give PT a fair trial after accepting the utility of exercises in stretching the muscles relaxed by USGDN. But after one month she was in the same situation and said that she would rather swim than do the exercises. She discontinued all exercises and after a week she came back with a smile on her face. Apparently, she knew her body better than anyone else and allowing her to follow her body wisdom proved to be the right formula for her. But the fact remained that she did exercise and stretch, albeit in a different form. She completed the USGDN sessions for another month. Some months later she had a bad fall and required USGDN for those pains. She has remained comfortable since, over the past 10 years. Elderly people, who have had an active lifestyle but have never done any formal 'exercise' find that their muscles may not take kindly to a sudden unaccustomed activity. Therefore, it's important to be open to the patient's input regarding the effectiveness of exercises, but only after they have diligently attempted them, under supervision.

How do you always needle the most painful points? Most patients ask this question. Actually, one has to simply target the muscles based on the anatomy whether a patient complains of pain in that area or not. There is an uncanny correlation between what the patients feel as pain and the sensations elicited by USGDN of the muscles involved in causing pain.

2. Electrical modalities in physiotherapy

These include transcutaneous electrical nerve stimulation (TENS), interferential current treatment (IFT), ultrasound massage, Laser and Stimpod. All these treatments temporarily relax the muscles through different mechanisms. Laser and Stimpod are particularly effective for initial symptomatic pain relief before starting definitive treatments. All patients first receive TENS or IFT to relax the muscles followed by the application of EMLA (known as prilox in India) cream, a specially compounded eutectic mixture of two local anaesthetics, lignocaine and prilocaine, which effectively numbs the skin before USGDN.

3. Myofascial release procedures

In simple terms, this is targeted massage, but physical therapists who specialize in its many different techniques can produce excellent results. We use a simple anatomical release of the muscles that resist needle passage and demonstrate LTRs during USGDN.

Yoga and chronic pain

Yoga comes from the root *Yuj* (unite) in the Sanskrit language, meaning a union of the body-mind-consciousness complex with the universal consciousness. The ancient Indian sages, the *rishi*s, discovered that focusing attention on sustained physical postures (called *asana*s), with continuous breath awareness, concentration on the various permutations and combinations of breathing (called *pranayama*) help to withdraw the mind from its constant chatter, still the constant meanderings of the mind and direct it towards quietude. The stilled and calm mind automatically turns inward for spiritual pursuits.

Briefly, yoga *asana*s are a very sophisticated and complex manipulation of muscles, firmly grounded in anatomy (study of the body structure). *Pranayamic* practices are a veritable treasure trove of physiological (study of bodily functions) information on the cardiorespiratory system. The sheer variety of manipulations of inspiration, expiration, and the pauses that come between the two are mind-boggling. The *rishi*s who formulated yoga as systematically organized psychophysical practices combined with breath control for stilling the mind to cultivate inner awareness, had an astounding mastery of both anatomy and physiology as is taught in modern medical curricula. The various techniques developed to manipulate the autonomic nervous system can, and do, form the basis of an autonomic workout that is exclusive to yoga and is unparalleled by any other practice in modern medicine. The currently popular studies and practices in 'Mindfulness' are ingrained practices of Yoga.

The exclusive purpose of yoga is spirituality but the same practices of *asana*s, *pranayama*, and mindfulness that quieten the mind are also immensely useful in pain, stress management, anger control, and psychiatric disorders. They automatically reduce the impulse traffic in the pain pathway to address the 'psycho' part of the biopsychosocial approach of modern pain management.

The fact that the mind directly controls the muscles is of paramount importance to the Ashirvad approach, and selected yogic practices are taught as an integral part of the treatment to target the mind-body connection in pain. It might entail adapting certain *asana*s or *mudra*s (subtle physical movements or sustained poses) as a part of physiotherapy to recruit, stretch, or strengthen the deconditioned muscles and use of awareness/mindfulness during the *asana*s or *pranayamic* practices to calm the mind.

Our exercise protocol put together with corroboration between expert physiotherapists and yoga experts, incorporates gentle *yogasana*s (stretching exercises). It comprises:

- First-stage exercises/*asana*s, gentle enough for severe pain conditions.
- Second-stage exercises/*asana*s for those enroute to recovery.
- Third-stage exercises for those who have completely recovered.

To have an indepth understanding in real time on how this protocol could influence or affect the spinal canal, the *asana*s were performed while the MRI was being recorded. Holding the spine twisted or bent or lifted steadily for four-to-five minutes can be quite strenuous! The body, accustomed to holding the posture for one minute in a yoga class, starts trembling and thus interfering with the quality of the MRI image capture. Despite these difficulties, this endeavour confirmed that the

Ashirvad protocol had positive effects on the spine. Only one posture, called 'bridging', was discarded as it tended to narrow the spinal canal.

After the patients recover and are well accustomed to the advanced-level exercises, they are advised to learn yoga with a formally trained yoga teacher, who follows the basic yoga dictum that an *asana* should be pleasurable and held steady without trembling. Pain patients with serious muscle imbalances have to be guided gently, always within their limits of flexibility. Once the patients settle down with regular exercising and yoga, they don't need further treatment. The only condition where a patient is immediately introduced to yoga is trigeminal neuralgia, which affects the face, mouth, teeth, and tongue and the muscles involved in speaking, chewing, and swallowing (masticatory muscles). Physiotherapy hardly has any specific exercises for the masticatory muscles, but yoga *mudra*s do specifically address them.[1]

The hazards of self-styled yoga

Yoga appears deceptively simple but actually, it is a complex science and is certainly not a panacea to be learnt online or by looking at a book or from YouTube videos. Good yoga teachers are, by their training, cautious, and they never teach advanced poses to a beginner. Only after the student is adept with milder *asana*s will they graduate to more complex postures. An unqualified person, whose brashness has not been tempered by formal training, cannot be a teacher and will definitely cause more damage than good. Discussed here are cases of some patients who suffered because of self-professed, cowboy-style personal trainers who seemed to think that yoga means vigorous physical contortions.

Weight-loss hazard: A 19-year-old girl developed a prolapsed lumbar 4–5 disc after 300 repetitions of an exercise called, "wall climbing" as guided by a personal trainer, in an endeavour to lose weight. At the age of 14 she had been treated at Ashirvad for migraine with PRF and USGDN. It was appalling to see in the MRI that the disc was occupying almost two-third of the spinal canal, making her bedridden, with severe shooting pain down the leg on sitting or standing. Several spine surgeons had advised surgery. Despite advice that she would not get back to normalcy with conservative treatment, she remained adamant and asserted, "Doctor, you reversed my migraine; you helped my father avoid disc surgery for his neck once and for back problems again.

I want you to try and help me avoid surgery." Finally, an epidural steroid injection gave her enough relief enabling her to sit up in bed. Thereafter, she would travel in an ambulance for USGDN, and soon enough she could stand and walk without pain for 10 minutes but travelling by public transport to college for classes on the second floor was out of the question. This made her agree for surgery after which she could walk 15 minutes without any problem. Unfortunately, four days later the disc prolapse recurred, requiring a repeat surgery. From there on it was a rapid downhill course for her. A spine fixation surgery did not help, nor did the third and fourth surgeries, done endoscopically. Her pains were back with redoubled ferocity and worse still, one leg got paralysed. She became three-times her original size due to repeated steroids given to reduce the inflammation after each surgery and lack of physical activity. The fifth surgery relieved her pain but at a very high cost: she lost bowel and bladder control. This was a very unfortunate tragic outcome for a young girl who went to a personal trainer to lose weight but instead, lost the vitality of her life. Neither she nor her wonderful family deserved to suffer this way because of someone else's callousness.

Disc prolapse after yoga: Mrs P was an obese homemaker in her early fifties with a protuberant belly. She went to some yoga trainer to lose weight, where she was subjected to brisk yoga in an attempt to convert yoga into an aerobic exercise! Although generally active with housework and social life, she had never 'exercised'. She lacked the good abdominal tone essential to maintain a healthy back. She was a disaster waiting to happen and she sustained acute lumbar 4–5 disc prolapse. She was in severe pain with shocks going down to her ankles despite medications, a complete bed rest for two weeks, and lumbar traction in a hospital for 15 days. However, an X-ray-guided transforaminal epidural steroid injection, USGDN, and Ashirvad exercises, particularly to strengthen the abdominal muscles, helped her resume her normal active life.

Cowboy personal trainers and random yoga for fitness: Ms N, a management executive in her early thirties, reported severe neck pain radiating to the left arm after 'yoga' done that morning with a personal trainer from a website, ostensibly to cure frequent neck pains. She had never done yoga before though she exercised occasionally in the gym and had run the Delhi half marathon once. Unbelievably, she had been made to do something like a *halasana* (the plough pose) repeatedly and rapidly by rocking herself from a lying down position to taking her legs over and behind her head and immediately returning to the supine pose. *Halasana* (Figure 45), is an advanced *asana*, not for beginners, however fit they might claim to be. It is taught only after the student has developed enough abdominal core muscle strength. It is done slowly, pausing at each step to focus on breathing. Most importantly, there is no concept of doing yoga 'rapidly'! Making a novice get in and out of *halasana* rapidly was extremely irresponsible. She was very lucky that she did not break her neck! Trained gymnasts perform such exercises, but they spend hours developing the requisite core muscle strength. Ironically, Ms N had started yoga to relieve her neck pains! USGDN done after neuromodulator and analgesic anti-inflammatory medication, showed serious spasms of the neck muscles but made her comfortable enough to get an MRI. She wanted to travel to attend a meeting in another metro city the next morning. But it was mandatory to get a MRI to rule out an acute disc prolapse before she travelled anywhere. It was almost certain that inflammation would set in soon to make her pain much worse. Predictably, the MRI showed an annular tear in the protruded cervical 5–6 disc.

An epidural steroid injection followed by six USGDN sessions relieved most of the pains. Since she was planning to travel to the US to join her husband, ultrasound guided Botox injected into her neck muscles

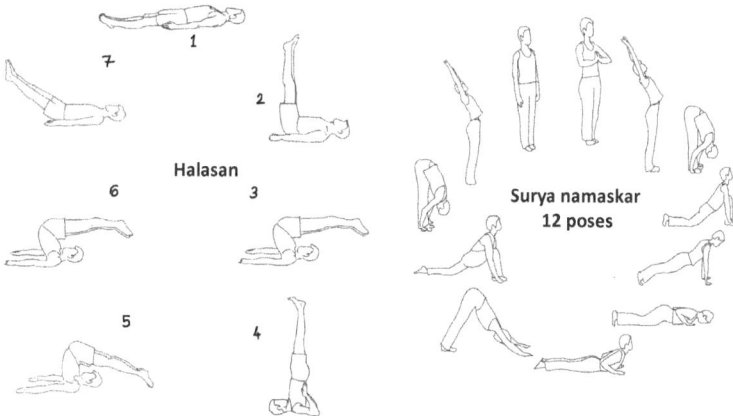

Figure 45. Serial poses of Halasana(left) and Suryanamaskar (right).

completely resolved her problems. She has remained pain-free with an active life for the past five years. All these expensive treatments apart from the suffering became necessary because of the distorted abuse of yoga. The trainer tried to brazenly abrogate himself of any responsibility by claiming none of his other clients had any problems!

Reference

[1] Vas, L., S. Phanse, K.S. Pawar et al. 2023. Ultrasound-guided dry needling of masticatory muscles in trigeminal neuralgia—A case series of 35 patients. J. Postgrad. Med. 69: 11–20.

Chapter 7

The Mind-Body Connection and Pain

Stress is a ubiquitous phenomenon of modern lifestyle with its high expectations, the wish to make an 'impact', or succeed, and the race for instant gratification. It has been held responsible for inducing diabetes, high blood pressure, heart disease, and hyperacidity, among others. That stress can exaggerate and aggravate various pains in the body is less understood, although the pains are as real as diabetes and heart disease. Unfortunately, pain cannot be measured like blood pressure or blood sugar. MRI, PET scans, or even the most modern and highly sophisticated blood tests are still too primitive to detect, let alone measure the subtle changes in the body-mind complex that produce pain. A functional MRI may validate the presence of pain but cannot quantify it. Interestingly, sonography demonstrates an association between severe pain and recordable spontaneous twitches in painful muscles at rest. These twitches increase on introducing needles for USGDN, and correspond with a steep increase in the patient's pain. In extremely painful conditions like CRPS, neuropathic pains, or even severe sprains, introducing the needle can provoke a LTR frenzy. But after 20 to 25 minutes, the twitches stop and so does the pain after the needle is removed. Therefore, an ultrasound can make pain 'visible', quantify it as 'severe', and ultimately provide a demonstration of pain relief. In less severe pains, twitches are absent in the resting muscle but introducing the needle provokes LTRs. In milder pains the needle triggers few, mild, twitches. Pain relief after USGDN, however, is invariably constant. These are *de novo* findings in the past 10 years and published as our cutting edge research. Since USGDN provides a treatment that authenticates the presence of pain as well as its relief in black and white, we rarely if ever, dismiss any patient's pain.

Chronic pain patients go doctor-shopping without getting relief

Multiple-doctor contact is the hallmark of a difficult medical problem. Chronic pain patients routinely go to many doctors in search of elusive relief. Whether depression causes pain or vice versa has been the subject of historic debate. Most pain patients know that they are suffering from actual pain and they get offended by the mere suggestion of underlying depression or anxiety and much more so at the mention of a psychological or psychiatric consultation.

Pain, the oldest human symptom, gave birth to medicine but medical practitioners neglect it as a mere signpost to an underlying disease. The perspective of the medical fraternity on pain remains an intricate enigma, often triggering debates, occasionally embodying conflicting viewpoints, and regrettably, exhibiting aspects of both hypocrisy and double standards. In certain cases, it even reflects outright complacency and lack of awareness. It is the hands-on experience and empathy of the doctor, which determines how much of the patient's history is heard with an open mind, acknowledged, and addressed.

Fortunately, the growing awareness of pain management has enabled urban patients to access pain clinics for proper treatment. However, some patients still encounter challenges in getting a proper diagnosis, leading them to consult multiple doctors and undergo numerous unnecessary investigations and treatments. There are several factors contributing to this situation.

Physician factors responsible for the situation

As recently as a few decades ago, chronic pain was dismissed with patronizing blitheness as purely psychological. But today it is an established fact that chronic pain is a disease, albeit one that has defied attempts at logical understanding and explanation.

The single-most important problem is the perspective of the doctor looking at a pain patient. Every doctor treats pain fairly commonly and as such, has a sense of familiarity with it without really understanding related intricacies. Acute pain is unequivocally acknowledged, empathized with, and promptly treated by most physicians. However, the attitude towards chronic pain is one of perplexed scepticism and few have the expertise to go into its depth.

For the longest time, chronic pain has not been objectively scrutinized from the patient's perspective. Few are the consultants even today, who look at chronic pain with scientific curiosity. Cursory prescription of painkillers and a referral to physiotherapy completes their limit of dealing with pain. This is neither callousness nor lack of concern; it is the case of doctors dealing with an enigma (albeit unwelcome), which does not fall within the purview of their specialty. This is similar to the description of an elephant by five blind men (Figure 46).

Surgical specialists (general surgeon, orthopaedic surgeon, neurosurgeon, or a gynaecologist) have an action-based outlook and place the emphasis on "What do I do?" They look at pain as something to be "cut out" and often their textbooks justify surgical interventions for relieving pain.

Medical specialists in the fields of neurology, rheumatology, and internal medicine among others, consist of thinkers of the medical profession. They have put forth theories and hypotheses about how drugs interrupt the pain pathway at various levels. They look at pain as something to be "drugged out" of the patient's system. Psychiatrists and psychologists focus on "counselling/drugging pain out of the psyche".

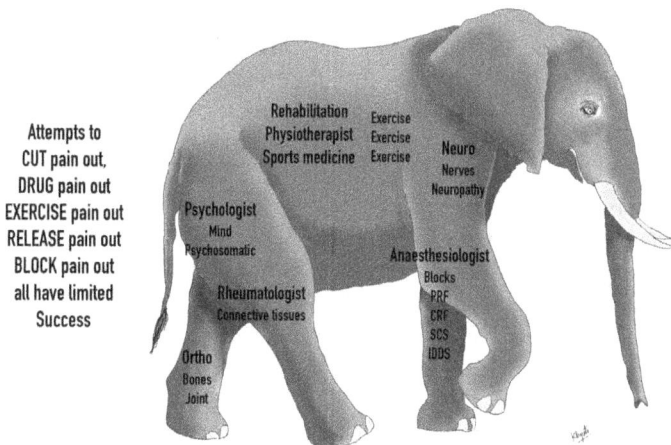

Figure 46. The doctors are the five blind men and chronic pain the elephant.

All these specialists try to fit chronic pain into the framework of their own specialty, viewing it through the telescope of each specialty to formulate possible treatments. Therefore, pain around the knee seems to come from the knee joint to an orthopaedic surgeon because joint replacement is his forte. When initial trials of pain killers, glucosamine supplements (presumed to improve cartilage health), physiotherapy or a hyaluron injection for knee lubrication, don't decrease the patient's pain/disability, joint replacement becomes the definitive treatment. An arthroscopy surgeon would automatically suggest an arthroscopic lavage of the knee, or stem-cell injection. If the knee pain is because of rheumatoid disease, the patient will be given disease-modifying antirheumatic drugs (DMARDs) to reduce the disease intensity and retard its progression, taking pain relief for granted. Unfortunately, long-standing rheumatic pains acquire neuromyopathic overtones and persist despite DMARDs. The same pain, therefore, is treated differently by different specialists with different perspectives. To a pain specialist, pain is the focus and will be primarily managed. Chronic pain is not confined to any one specialty; it spans across specialties and is best managed by a multidisciplinary approach combining pain relief along with treatment of its cause.

Pain specialists are anaesthesiologists, who combine surgical and medical attitudes of 'doing' and 'thinking'. They are in their element when working with their hands but have to develop very focussed thinking to steer the patient safely through the complex dynamics of anaesthesia. The title, peri-operative physician, describes their ability to foresee the myriad problems that can arise when they manipulate the physiology of the heart, brain, and kidney while administering anaesthesia.

However, pain specialists are late entrants into the field of chronic pain. Most, if not all, thought processes and concepts ingrained in pain management have come from pioneers from orthopaedics, neurology, or rheumatology. Pain specialists simply inherited prevailing theories and hypotheses on pain and focussed on "blocking out" pain by devising more and more sophisticated interventional treatments for the nerves and joints predesignated as the causes of pain. As a result, contemporary treatments in pain management address pain from the historic perspectives of orthopaedics, neurology, and rheumatology. But the catch in this approach is that pain management was born as a separate specialty only because nerve- and joint-centric thought processes were quasi-effective!

Actually, a radically different approach is needed: A clear understanding of what causes different pains, how they express themselves, the limitations that the patients may feel in directing the doctor's attention to their suffering, and most importantly, how to relieve it. We believe that our approach of listening to patients and letting them guide our understanding of pain is the first step in the right direction. Over the years, this new patient-centric understanding of pain has revealed different perspectives and changed the concepts of the cause and effect of pain. Current practices have therefore, to be changed from nerve-centric treatments to include a nerve + joint + muscle-centric approach for achieving success with a holistic body-mind approach to explain the enigma of pain.

Very clearly, it is not just the pain that bothers patients; the inability to do the routine things that they were doing so easily earlier, distresses them more. Once they are able to perform their daily duties after treatment, they regain their self-esteem and confidence about their usefulness to the family and society and get on with their lives.

Patient factors responsible for the perpetuation of chronic pain

*Unrealistic expectation*s: Patients feel that expensive treatments must produce great and almost instant results and since they have come to a pain specialist, they should get immediate and 100 per cent relief. Mental attitudes play a pivotal role in dissatisfaction.

Passive recipients: Patients expect the doctor to provide miraculous relief while they remain passive, without assuming any responsibility for getting better, for changing their attitude towards life in general, and pain in particular. They have limited compliance to medication, physiotherapy, pacing themselves to avoid pain, and coping with unavoidable limitations. Chronic pain responds better to co-contributors than to passive recipients.

Internet-educated patients from privileged backgrounds: The wealth of information on the Internet requires an ability for discriminative reading between the lines for an educated and prudent understanding. Across-the-board generalized information, far removed from ground reality can be misleading. Many patients read up extensively, use superficially gathered medical terminology to describe their problems, dropping names of overseas doctor just to convey that their problem has baffled even 'foreign' experts. They are convinced that their problems are unique, and no doctor will ever solve it and go doctor-shopping. Unless they come down to *terra firma*, and accept that the doctor is on their side, they are unlikely to improve.

Degenerative effects of age necessitate regular treatment: Treatments can successfully reverse pain but cannot stall the relentless ageing process. Jokingly, one can say that if it were possible to reverse the clock and become ten years younger, then it would be possible to be pain-free without medication! Realistically, just as greying hair requires regular colouring, the body with its ageing creaky joints and stiff muscles requires regular exercise, medications or USGDN or neural interventions as and when necessary.

Pain medications are necessary: Indian patients have no problem in taking their diabetes, blood pressure, and heart medications for a lifetime but believe that pain medication should be stopped at the first opportunity (despite repeated advice to the contrary); that these are unnecessary, harmful, weakening, and addictive. Pain medicines are often stopped just to check if the pain has vanished, or to sceptically wonder, for how long should anyone have to take painkillers? And finally, there is the resigned conclusion that the pain has not really gone but is only suppressed by medicines. They want a single dose to provide permanent pain relief! Pain medicines provide relief and pave the way to an active and normal life, but they need consistent follow-up. Most patients continue to use, overuse, misuse, and even perhaps abuse, the body almost on an hourly, daily basis; naturally there will be injuries to the structures that are already weakened by the degenerative effects of ageing. One needs to take judicious care of the body to get the maximum out of it. Not only patients, but many doctors, unfamiliar with pain management, don't understand that regular medications are necessary for the constant control of chronic pain and abrupt cessation of pain medications can result in a major backlash.

A related case study: An 80-year-old lady with MPS and lumbar canal stenosis, was well-controlled on a regular low dose of tramadol-paracetamol combination and night-time pregabalin. Unfortunately, she developed a mild heart attack but with a good ejection fraction (percentage of blood pumped out of heart with each contraction) of 45 per cent was admitted to an ICU for observation.

The treating physician put her on cardiac medications but stopped the pain medications. The old lady, already worried and distressed, spending the night in unfamiliar surroundings and more importantly, deprived of the pain medications, which routinely sedated her mildly and controlled her pains, complained bitterly about body pains and a sleepless night. The heightened cardiac workload from increased heart rate and blood pressure made her mild attack become severe overnight with considerable myocardial damage and a lowered ejection fraction (15 per cent). An emergency angioplasty salvaged the situation, but she continues with the borderline ejection fraction of 15 per cent, which has permanently restricted her daily activities and diminished her quality of life. Had her pain medications been continued, she might have recovered with minimum damage and a good ejection fraction.

Selective hearing: Patients will register only what they wish to hear. If they are told of "a possibility of the treatment reducing the pain," it is construed as a promise of eliminating pain! Explanations about the biopsychosocial nature of pain, and its recalcitrance due to ageing are simply filtered out or not registered.

The "half-empty glass" syndrome

The pain pathway in chronic pain has equal inputs from both the body and the mind. Anxiety, depression, suspicion, or frank disbelief in the ability of the doctor or treatment, or the whole medical system contributes to the poor response to pain treatments. Some patients carry a negative load on their minds, that their pain is so special and so weird that they have been singled out for suffering. They simply turn a deaf ear to the explanation that the mind turns negative in chronic pain because of the direct neural projection from the thalamus to the emotional areas of the brain (Figure 4, Chapter 1). They even get very offended at the very mention of a psychological consultation or at taking a verbal test like the Minnesota Multiphasic Personality Inventory (MMPI) that evaluates the contribution of the mind to the pain. Fortunately, most patients rise above negativity while a few nurture it.

Pain and disability are bodily inputs, which get addressed with mathematical precision by comprehensive targeting of all pain generators, nerves, muscles, joints. But to address the mind, the bond of confidence and trust between the doctor and patient is essential. Fortunately, a majority of the patients show this confidence and come to understand many things about themselves that they were hitherto unaware of. Of course, a patient's trust and confidence have to be earned by the doctor.

Matter over mind: At the other end of the spectrum are the patients for whom the cup is permanently half empty, who will remain defeated even if the pain is reduced. They know their pain is less but ignore the improvement. Their expectations are unrealistic because they want life to be as they have decided, "it should be". It is an impossible task to satisfy anyone who has a closed unrealistic mind.

When it is pointed out to that from a bedridden state, they are now mobile, independent, active, at a far lowered level of pain, they hesitate, with a petulant, almost reluctant admission that the pain is less, and there is increased activity on a daily basis, but there is always the plaintive cry, "*but* the pain is still there!" and "I want to be pain-free; I don't want pain medications!" Patients want to be pain-free and taken off medication. With this cup perennially in the half-empty category we can only succeed after they accept that their own mind can become their worst enemy; if they wish to do well, they need to make their mind their best friend.

On initial examination, it is impossible to know the contribution of the mind in reinforcing the pain. Some patients often stand at extreme poles. In between these two extremes lie all the other patients. Some are diffident but ready to be guided; some are disbelieving that they will ever get better but after being pleasantly surprised by some relief are ready to be guided; some are defiant but will eventually be guided, and yet others who are cautious, holding onto their pain till they convince themselves that it is definitely on the downswing. Needless to say, they need constant encouragement.

Mind over matter: Sometimes, after pain relief, a patient displays a complete *volte face* from being the depressed and disabled person to being the complete winner. They are upfront enough to let us do whatever is necessary to make them better, because they want to get back to a normal life.

The power of the mind: The road to recovery is a slow process of re-education about recovering from pain and more importantly, the recovery from disability. To comprehend the power of the mind, one only needs to reflect on the baffling finding that soldiers with serious wounds at the height of battle, have no pain! This is a fascinating insight of how the brain simply blocks off the pain signals to allow the soldier to fight and survive a potentially fatal situation and complain only after he is stabilized in a hospital. Conversely there is a situation where the mind intensifies pain instead of negating it, responding with emotions, fear, panic, and anxiety that actually amplify physical discomfort.

Attitude counts

The attitude of the patient is crucial, and in the final analysis, it is the patient who calls the shots and the pain physician can only be a facilitator. The following case studies specifically show the diverse impact of attitudes on the course of treatment and the consequent outcomes: ranging from negative and uncooperative, despondent and suicidal, and positive and care-free, faith working wonders, objective and down to earth, and all the shades of grey, black and white.

Negative and uncooperative: Ms P was a fifty-year-old, short obese homemaker, bedridden with pain despite two back surgeries. She reported 70 per cent pain relief after treatment at Ashirvad. However, her response was always a litany of, "I cant's, whys, and hows": "I just can't exercise; why physiotherapy? How long are pain medications to be taken? Why a psychologist? There is nothing wrong with my mind! I am tired going to so many hospitals...." and so on. She was told firmly that if she wished to get better, she had to continue treatment. She had a very supportive husband who was greatly relieved that his wife was finally comfortable, but he was helpless because she would get angry and sulk if he said anything. She stopped treatment with the excuse that pain management required too much work—take medicines, do exercise, and get USGDN! She ignored and dismissed the benefits of her regained abilities of morning walk and doing housework. This protest or negative reaction was coming from a patient who had been completely bedridden! Because of her state of denial she chose to condemn herself to a lifetime of unnecessary limitations.

Pain and suffering

Dame Cicely Saunders coined the term "total pain", to acknowledge that pain has physical, psychological, social, emotional, and spiritual components that affect a person's pain experience. The "total pain" (Figure 47) experience is specific to each patient's particular situation. Therefore, to treat pain effectively, a bio (physical), psycho (mind,

Physical, Psychological, Social & Spiritual Pains

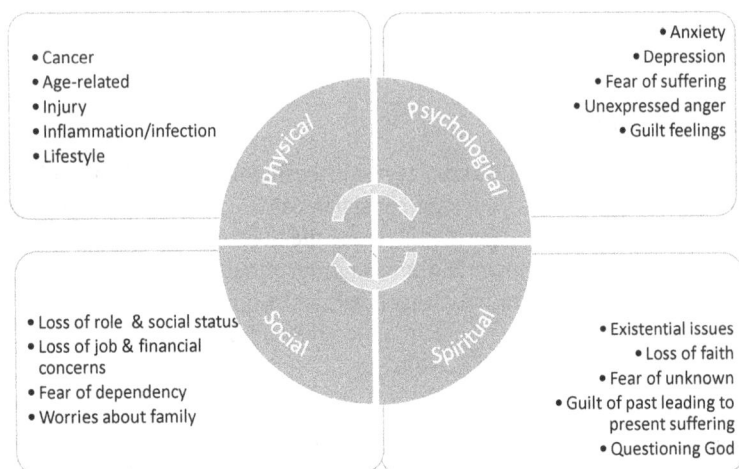

- Cancer
- Age-related
- Injury
- Inflammation/infection
- Lifestyle

- Anxiety
- Depression
- Fear of suffering
- Unexpressed anger
- Guilt feelings

- Loss of role & social status
- Loss of job & financial concerns
- Fear of dependency
- Worries about family

- Existential issues
- Loss of faith
- Fear of unknown
- Guilt of past leading to present suffering
- Questioning God

Figure 47. Total pain.

emotion, spiritual), and social (societal status, role loss, job loss, financial concerns, fear of dependency, family worries) approach is essential. The spiritual concerns like existential issues, loss of faith, fear of the unknown, past guilt leading to present suffering, and questioning God, become important in palliative care.

There are consequences of being in constant pain, which changes the physiology of the nerves, the spinal cord, and the brain. Chronic pain interferes with cognition and attention; it causes emotional distress, feelings such as unexpressed anger, hopelessness, frustration, sadness, anxiety, and depression and all of these collectively interfere with daily-life activities. These emotions negatively affect relationships and interpersonal interactions. They sap the energy and certainly make the person feel unwell. The more severe the pain, the heavier the toll it takes on the person's well-being. The negative emotions of fear, depression, stress, and anxiety compound the intensity or prolong the pain. However, it is rare that pain originates from a purely psychological condition (psychogenic pain).

In a spiritual black hole of a dark mind: Mr R, aged 48, had a history of recurrent anal pain for six years after repeated surgery for haemorrhoids and fissures. He had gone through a difficult divorce. Unfortunately,

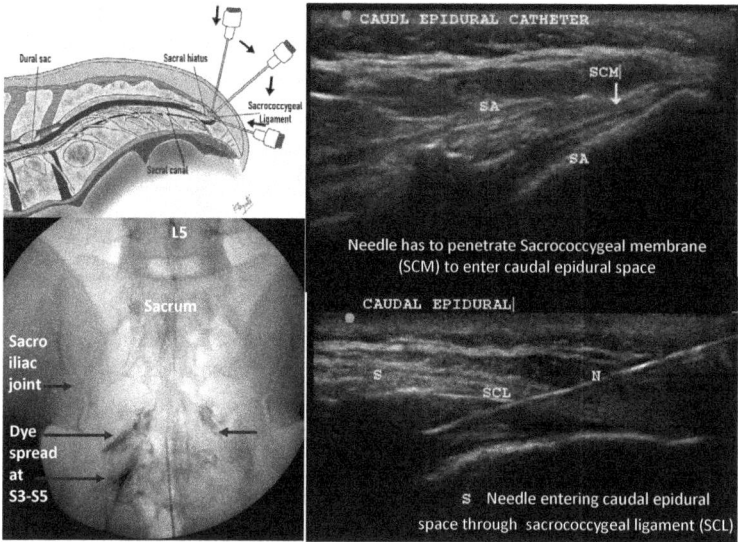

Figure 48. Top left: Section diagram of sacrum (SA). Right: Sonography of lower sacrum showing sacrococcygeal membrane (SCM). Bottom left: Dye spread around S2-5 nerves. Right: Needle (N) entering caudal epidural space.

the last surgery had left him with severe chronic neuropathic pain. He was bedridden, completely demoralized, and in deep depression. It was obvious that first and foremost, he needed to see a psychiatrist and he promised that he would as soon as his pain was controlled and he was mobile. After CNB with caudal catheter (Figure 48) and Botox, he improved steadily for a week and was comfortable but then the problems started. Unreasonably, he insisted that the catheter be removed prematurely because he could not tolerate the intestinal gurgling caused by antibiotics. Adamantly, he was not ready to try a change in the antibiotics. The catheter was removed before achieving complete pain relief. However, with USGDN he improved and could walk 30 minutes, twice daily, and became self-sufficient for his daily activities. At every visit however, the refrain was that he was miserable, what if the pain came back? The psychiatrist and the psychologist, to whom he was sent for this catastrophizing, also complained that he was not following up with them after the first consultation. His justification was that they were unable to help him and that their medicines caused confusion and constipation. Thus, he saw no point in continuing. Suggestions that he take up a job to occupy the devil's workshop that his mind had become, fell on deaf ears. His argument was that he was financially well off and had no need to work. He was not close to any friends or relatives. He refused such options as electroconvulsive therapy for the depression or seek solace in spirituality. His stock response was that he saw no purpose in continuing. He was planning to end his life through the Dignitas Foundation of Switzerland, a country that allows euthanasia. Mr M stated quite matter-of-factly that this non-profit organization provides physician-assisted ending. Even his father's agonized appeal to desist failed. This individual had set his goal on euthanasia, which he pursued relentlessly to its very tragic end. It is terribly disheartening when a patient refuses to acknowledge the power of extreme negativity of the mind and the games it can play. This state of denial can only be breached when the patient allows the doctor 'in'. Thinking of this tormented soul, as a doctor one realizes how powerless or helpless one is when the patient forbids entry. It was not just the pain that he wanted to end, but it was his life itself that he wanted to end.

This case study emphasizes how a negative mind inexorably pursues its nihilistic goals, impervious to the feelings of those left behind. The old father has to live with the terrible reality and with the rankling question, 'Why?' Why did his intelligent son, who had ticked every box of success in modern-day life, choose to exit life this way?

Thankfully, there is a flip side to the coin, opposite to this dismal and dark view. And there are plenty of heartening cases, as a majority of patients do readily accept the help available (Chapter 8).

Fibromyalgia

FM patients are in a class by themselves because of their youth, intelligence, and sensitivity coupled with highly disabling pain. FM is called a central excitation syndrome because the pain pathway in CNS appears to be in a state of perpetual excitation. The mind is but a part of the CNS and its excitation mirrors that of the CNS. These people benefit from medication, gentle physiotherapy and myofascial release but keep developing new pains. Strategically timed PRF, USGDN and Botox can be very useful to keep them going. Returning to a job is the best therapy but then it takes coping strategies, an acceptance of FM and the efficacy of the above treatments to get them there. Several patients have successfully completed the uphill task of understanding the two-way traffic between their active minds troubled by painful bodies.

Each one of them has figured out just how best to pace his/her daily activities so as to cope with FM and regain control over their lives.

Ms RS: At the first consultation, Ms RS was despondent at her inability to do simple activities like waking up comfortably in the morning, bathing, and dressing. Work was out of the question because of the pain. She was very angry with life in general, with herself, and she was, understandably, furious and bitter with some doctors for implying that her pain was more in her head. She was reassured to learn that often chronic pain is more because of, "What's *not* in the doctor's head rather than the pain being in the patient's head." She accepted the diagnosis of fibromyalgia and the course of treatment that could support her to set up a realistic, feasible target for activities and work towards it till she was satisfied. She and her supportive husband decided to have PRF, Botox, and USGDN for the various pains she was experiencing. Over the course of five to six months she gradually increased her activities with most of her pains at acceptable levels. She understood the need to go slow, listen to her body, and how not to listen to the monkey, that was her mind. With all this her natural empathetic vibrant personality re-emerged over the next six months and she started volunteering with elders. Thereafter she gradually tapered her treatment but remains in touch.

Hearing about "What's *not* in the doctor's head ...." had the honourable Shri SM Krishna, the then Governor of the State of Maharashtra, highly amused. He had sought treatment for an unusual sensation of the ground being wavy beneath his feet. During his public appearances as part of his official responsibilities, he had to walk very gingerly to avoid imbalance. As the Governor, he had at his disposal a galaxy of eminent doctors yet, the solution to this problem had remained elusive. While his wife was being treated for fibromyalgia, he had casually spoken about his problem and was surprised when USGDN was suggested as a treatment for it. He was curious about the rationale behind the suggestion of USGDN of the neck muscles as a treatment—the body posture and stance are determined by non-stop inputs from the Golgi tendon organs from the neck muscles and the semi-circular canals in the inner ear, which act like the spirit level used by stonemasons to build their walls straight. The semi-circular canals sense the body posture to know how the body is poised, bent forward or backward, or sideways so that the cerebellum and the motor areas of the brain involved in maintaining posture can make the necessary adjustments to maintain balance. The information system is so accurate that any loss of balance is corrected instantaneously by 'righting' the reflexes, which are mediated by the muscles that maintain posture and stance in the leg, back, and trunk. However, neck muscles shortened by MTrPs can fix the neck in subtly abnormal positions, stressing the Golgi tendon organs, and tilting the semi-circular canals to feed misinformation to the complex mechanisms that balance the body. As a result, the person can feel a sense of vertigo, giddiness, floating, or that the ground is wavy. Systematic USGDN of the neck de-stresses the Golgi tendon organs, relaxes the muscles, so that they can hold the head up in a normal position. This explanation seemed to fascinate Mr Krishna and he readily agreed for USGDN. After three-four sessions of needling, he was no longer unsure about where the ground was and he regained his normal confident stride. He commented, "The improvement is really remarkable! Just a few needles in my neck and my limitations have completely disappeared, wonderful treatment!" His relief and happiness were discernible that such a perplexing problem could be eliminated so easily.

Enjoyed her pain: Ms K in her late 30s was limping because of groin pain and had seen several doctors, taken many treatments for various pains in the neck, chest, back, and extremities. She had stopped working three years earlier and was financially dependent on her aged parents. Ms K's detailed and intricate history, embellished with many technical terms of pain and even the names of most of her muscles, was intriguing as if she was almost enjoying her pain! Her MRI was pristine and other investigations normal. She improved well with PRF of the hip and groin nerves and USGDN of the lower limb muscles. But the delight in describing every little symptom continued. By now there were no pains, so it was more of, "stiffness in my quads when I do this stretch, or my adductors pull when I stretch this way... and so on." On the topic of returning to a job, she would be evasive and give various excuses, "I have not worked for three years; no one will give me a job that I deserve; I can't travel, so I have to compromise a lot on salary if I take a job near my house; I have a lot of work at home...." Fortunately, she accepted the frank and direct advice that she really had too much time on her hands, so her mind was forever searching like a radar, looking for issues in the body. Additionally, her idle mind would continue to keep wandering round and round, almost seeking problems within the body and mind. It was gently pointed out to her that her aged parents, were equally worried about her sitting at home, and being financially dependent on them.

Despite the involvement with her bodily issues, she was quite amenable to these suggestions and finally, took up a job on the condition that she could continue a fortnightly review at the clinic to ensure her fitness. She required this support for another 6 to 8 months. Five years later, she has transformed into an independent and gainfully employed woman taking care of her parents.

On an optimistic note, the concept of treating neuromyopathy with PRF for nerves, ultrasound guided Botox and needling for muscles along with necessary lifestyle changes, addresses the body. The mind with its attitudes plays a key role and is treated by the doctor-patient partnership, which makes a successful reversal of many terrible pain conditions possible. It becomes the physicians' job to nudge the patient in the right direction, point out that an approach with hope, positive attitude and a willingness to change is more conducive to pain relief. The Ashirvad experience is rife with stories of patients who have frequently demonstrated the power and resilience of the human mind.

Chapter 8
Case Studies

Much of the pain management journey has been a process of on-the-job learning, involving understanding, treatment, and learning—from the pains, sorrows, and joys experienced by the patients.

Cancer pain patients

Cancerous growth invades, damages, and compresses the nerves in its vicinity or starves the tissue (including nerves) of adequate blood supply to cause ischaemic pain. Additionally, surgery, radiation, and chemotherapy cause neuromyopathy. Thus, nerves/muscles get intimately involved in generating, maintaining, and transmitting cancer pain. Neuromodulators influence the electrochemical events in pain transmission in the PNS and CNS with a profound effect in pain reduction.

A humbling experience

One of first unique case studies, which became educational was Ms B, with terminal mandible (lower jawbone) cancer. She was extremely restless, unable to sleep or even think coherently with severe head and face pain, unresponsive to morphine. The simple introduction of pregabalin brought down the pain by 50 per cent. Once pain patients know that there is someone who can possibly help them, they latch on to that doctor and demand more and continuing relief, providing a great opportunity for the pain physician to achieve unexpected results. After the initial euphoria of being able to sleep and eat well, she said, "Do whatever you want but my pain should go away." Head, face and neck, pains relay in the stellate ganglion and an SGB (Chapter 3,

Figure 18) reduced her residual pain immediately and significantly but Ms B was yet to be satisfied. She did not like the drowsiness, nausea, and the constipation associated with morphine. Reducing the dosage brought some of the pains back. Suspecting her pains to be coming from the muscles, which appeared to be in extremely severe spasm, DN of the face, head, and the neck muscles was performed. While the thought of needles seems unpleasant, most patients find that the needling produces 'good', or "relieving pain", which is followed by dramatic reduction of the original pain. Ms B was no different and continued to be pain-free till she died a month later, unbeholden to pain or a mind befuddled by opioid drugs.

This near total comfort for a terminal cancer patient became possible with the combination of medication+SGB+DN. Muscle pain is a very important but little-known aspect of head-neck cancer pain. This experience and others thereafter led to the eventual understanding of neuromyopathy. The concept of muscle involvement in cancer pain is not really understood even today despite the publication of our results and presentations at conferences (Chapter 2 references 3, 4, and 12–15).

Ms HS—Positivity in death: An alarmed psychiatrist was at his wits end because his paediatrician wife had asked for help to end her life. Her terminal ovarian cancer had progressed despite repeated surgeries, chemotherapy, and radiation. HS was in a state of confusion from excruciating back and thigh pain from metastases in the lumbar plexus of nerves that supplies the thigh, unrelieved severe colic, and opioids (oral morphine+intramuscular tramadol injection+50 micrograms fentanyl patch). She was crawling all over her bed in a darkened room in a futile attempt to find a comfortable position. After thorough examination and discussion, a test injection of 0.3 mg morphine into her CSF the next day gave good relief. The subsequent day a morphine intrathecal pump was implanted into her abdomen (Figure 27, Chapter 2). Continuous infusion of 0.48 mg/day morphine (< 1/300 of her oral dose) and clonidine made her totally pain-free without the constipation and nausea from oral morphine, tramadol, and fentanyl. With this respite, she threw herself back into life with renewed vigour and started working part-time within three months. From being a person who wished to end her life she now had an ardent wish to prolong her life. She started chemotherapy with great hope and enthusiasm. Unfortunately, after three months she developed agranulocytosis (blood cell production shutdown) requiring dedicated barrier nursing care against infections and several blood transfusions for recovery. But without the chemotherapy control, her cancer started spreading. Escalating the morphine from 0.48 mg/day to 4 mg/day was not completely satisfactory. Based on the Indian experience of the safety of short-term intraspinal ketamine, the option (albeit off-label) of adding it to the pump was discussed. HS immediately gave completely trusting consent, adding an immense responsibility. The acid test in such situations always is, would one do the same for oneself and one's family, if the need arose? If the answer is yes, then one goes ahead. There was no data about the long-term safety of intrathecal ketamine but HS, had only a few weeks or months to live. Therefore, rather than worry about a theoretical risk, 4 mg/day ketamine was added. This kept her completely pain-free. Her indomitable spirit kept her going for another two months but the inexorable march of cancer claimed her with kidney failure. HS's battle exemplified Albert Schweitzer's quote, "Pain is a more terrible lord of mankind than even death himself," and his prayer, "...that I can save him from days of torture...is my great and ever new privilege." HS was gone but she left behind a dominant feeling of positivity.

Mr P—Can't deal with any more pain: Mr P had multiple myeloma with excruciating pains despite morphine, fentanyl, and neuromodulators. The referring doctor, a highly respected cardiothoracic surgeon and teacher knew that his childhood friend did not have long to live, but could anything be done for his immense suffering? Mr P could only speak in grunts: "I am exhausted, and I don't want to suffer any more. I have lived well, and I would like to go with dignity if you can help me." After a detailed discussion, he and his physiotherapist wife agreed for implanting the intrathecal pump.

The morphine test dose injection and the implanted pump provided very good pain relief. Although he became pain-free, it was explained to him that total pain relief with the advancing cancer was difficult and 70 to 80 per cent pain relief under the circumstances was more realistic He agreed, but said, "Doc, please do your best." He was very happy for five months but then mild pains restarted. Morphine pump patients get so used to the complete pain relief that they become intolerant of even very mild pains, turning a deaf ear to the explanations about realistic expectations. Increasing the morphine and clonidine (which enhances morphine action) doses necessitated frequent morphine refills. He was on oral morphine tablets and a fentanyl lollipop for the breakthrough pains that erupted despite intrathecal morphine. One day he called in panic with this catastrophizing, "Doc, I am not worried about death, I have settled all my affairs and have made my peace with my life's situations, but the thought of returning pain scares me. So please do something." He could be given ketamine, a very powerful pain killer anaesthetic. But his wife had to take the responsibility keeping it under lock and key and administering the specially prepared oral ketamine in correct dosage. Mrs P saw to it that her husband got the doses as needed. This gave him the zero-pain status that he desperately wanted. His next worry was what if he developed tolerance to oral ketamine as well. After the reassurance that we could increase ketamine and morphine doses indefinitely, he was relaxed and comfortable till the end.

The Paralysed shall walk!

Screaming lady: A patient SK was referred to us in 2004 for deafferentation pain and spasms in her paralysed lower limbs after decompression spine surgery for tuberculosis. The loss of sensory input into the CNS as in paralysis or total nerve damage causes this. She was called the "screaming lady" because of her screams when her lower limbs suddenly scissored into excruciatingly painful involuntary spasms, which continued unabated despite neuromodulator medication and baclofen, a muscle relaxant. A spinal test dose injection of baclofen into CSF produced a dramatic cessation of her painful spasms. She was very relieved and happy! But for a prolonged effect, minuscule baclofen doses (1/100 of oral dose) needed to be injected continuously through an implanted intrathecal pump, directly into CSF around the spinal cord, the place of origin of her muscle spasms.

But there was a practical problem. SK could not afford an intrathecal baclofen pump, which works only in CSF. Instead, the family consented to placing a catheter in the epidural space just outside the CSF. This was connected to an implanted port. Local anaesthetic and morphine injections from an external pump given through the skin into the port would flow into the epidural space, through the catheter (similar to Figure 26, Chapter 2). These drugs would still have access to the spinal cord, the final common pathway for all pains. Morphine would control the pain although not the spasms themselves. As expected, she was fairly comfortable despite continued spasms. Unfortunately, after three months, a catheter blockage put SK back to square one with severe spasms and continuous pains despite heavy oral opioids. There would be a crowd outside her ward complaining about how disruptive her screams were. Since their complaints were genuine and the complainants were themselves patients, one could empathize. But finally, it had to be said, "... she is a patient of this hospital coming from the same society as everyone here. She deserves sympathy for her agony despite maximum painkillers!"

SK could not survive this level of pain for long but how were we going to get an intrathecal pump that cost four lakhs? Fortunately, a company called Medtronic, sponsored a pump and wrote off the cost to educational expenses of demonstrating the implantation of an intrathecal pump in a neurology conference. The pump made a miraculous difference to both the pain and the patient's attitude! From the exhausted woman screaming with pain, lack of nutrition, and sleep—she was a new human being overnight, peacefully reading in her bed, like the calm person that she had been before the pain set in (Figure 27, Chapter 2).

Interestingly, two months later, there were exciting movement flickers in her feet and ankles. This meant she could possibly recover some movements! USGDN was started with the vague assumption that simultaneous contraction of all the lower limb muscles was immobilizing the whole limb mimicking a flaccid paralysis. By relieving the spasm, USGDN clearly confirmed the hypothesis that simultaneous contraction in opposing muscle groups were making movements impossible, giving an impression of paralysis. Gradually her movements improved till she could comfortably stand and walk around with callipers and a walker. Pain was a thing of the past! Regained ability to help with the housework boosted her self-esteem and made life meaningful. Her daughter, an OT nurse, learnt the technique of refilling the pump. Family support is wonderful and provides a very stable empowering base for people like SK to deal with adversity with the confidence that they don't have to face their predicament alone. SK was blessed with caring children who did their utmost to keep her happy and comfortable. After three years her pump stalled but by this time, with her resumed limb usage, the spasms and pains were no longer a major problem, and SK settled well on a low dose of oral morphine.

Doc, healing me is your responsibility! Mr DP, 73-year-old simple villager with this very straightforward expectation was carried into the clinic because of quadriplegia (paralysis of all four limbs) after a spinal cord injury. He had terrible burning pain all over the body that starts in the recovery phase from spinal cord injury (causalgia). After a SGB reduced the burning by half, his faith in the treatment and his desire to improve was so absolute that he fully expected to walk after the treatment.

He had no doubt that he would be cured. This kind of faith is scary because it demands a miraculous cure that may be medically impossible. But this implicit faith, by itself, also carries the patient forward to an unimaginable recovery. He was treated with the offbeat assumption that his inability to move was because opposing muscle groups were simultaneously contracting (abnormal co-contraction); the antagonist would contract with the agonist instead of relaxing and letting the agonist contract. This makes movement impossible mimicking paralysis. His limb muscles just recovering from complete paralysis, were intrinsically too weak to override the resistance of co-contraction. Targeted and regular USGDN followed-up by physiotherapy of agonist/antagonist combinations of the specific movements of all four limbs gradually restored his movements. In a span of eight weeks he was walking freely. He independently managed all his daily activities and worked with his son in the family's sawmill. This went on for seven years with USGDN at six-to-eight-month intervals and a few regular medications that he gracefully accepted. Interestingly, he would grumble and complain, but only in the clinic. After a little venting, he would go out and be cheerful. Enquiries with the family revealed that he never complained at home. A significant feature of the doctor-patient interaction is the patient's need to vent where they can be expected to be listened to with patience and empathy; express their innermost frustrations, fears and doubts.

DP was really the salt of the earth, simple, realistic and practical, with a childlike trust in the order of things. He had an abiding acceptance of circumstances which can be very empowering; one can live gracefully with a sense of unequivocal responsibility towards life even with quadriplegia complications. Living as a paralytic was unacceptable and giving up was not an option; so, he optimized the gifts life had granted him. DP passed away peacefully in his sleep at 80 years, but his benign simplicity, fortitude in the face of misfortune, and unconditional acceptance of life continues to enliven those who interacted with him.

Relieve my pain or give me poison! There are a few pain management situations as drastic as this. The chief cardiothoracic surgeon from a major teaching hospital of Mumbai and his ophthalmologist wife wanted treatment for her mother with severe shooting electrical shock-like pains down both her legs. The problem was that the old lady was in ICU for a mild heart attack but was extremely miffed with everyone because her worsening back pain of four months remained undiagnosed initially, and now the heart attack precluded the surgery, which had promised long awaited relief from spinal tuberculosis pain. The normally mild-mannered lady blew her top and delivered an ultimatum, "I can't bear this pain anymore. All you did was make me traipse around doctors, tests and now ICU! Either relieve my pain or give me poison to end my life!"

Surgery was too risky after the heart attack. Intravenously administered opioids and steroids remained ineffective. The doctor couple with all medical facilities at their disposal, were at their wits end trying to find a way out. The patient, tossing around in the bed to find even the slightest comfort from her severe distress was in a state of confusion. Could she be helped, and urgently?

The MRI showed tubercular destruction of the inflamed lumbar 4–5 intervertebral disc. To convince the lady, who was writhing in pain, to remain still even for the brief moment required for an X-ray guided block, required employing every possible form of persuasion. After identifying the dye spread at the L4–5 epidural space, a local anaesthetic and steroid triamcinolone was administered to reduce the disc inflammation, the root cause of the pain. Soon after the procedure, 'Ajji' (grandmother in the regional language, Marathi) was lying very still. On enquiry, looking rather disbelievingly, she said "I can't believe it! The 100 snakes with razor-sharp teeth constantly biting and chewing the flesh off, injecting burning poison", have stopped! Such was the graphic description of her pain, which elicited shudders all around.

A month later, her state was indeed pathetic. This indomitable lady, who had always presided over her household, cooking up a storm and feeding everyone, was lying paralysed and helpless unable to even feed herself. There was severe muscle loss with the fat hanging free without the anchoring effect of muscles. Her daughter found a young physiotherapist just discovering the pleasures of his profession, with enough time to spare for Ajji but there was only so much physiotherapy could do. Unfortunately, the heavy antitubercular drug doses caused jaundice necessitating withdrawal of all drugs till the liver recovered. Lack of the muscle-relaxing action of lyrica stiffened the muscle remnants bringing some of the pain back.

As her condition was reviewed it seemed that paralysis/weakness was probably because one spastic muscle group tethered the other, making movements impossible. Botox seemed the best course of treatment to relax the spastic muscles. Given the already paralysed state of her muscle, the suggestion of Botox was rather drastic. But the family reposed enough faith in the "magic" of pain management to repeat the original success. Fortunately, the therapy was spot on. Ajji and the physiotherapist were back in business! Soon enough, at another home visit, she proudly donned knee braces, called for her walker, and stood up, although trembling yet triumphantly acknowledging the standing ovation! Thereafter it was easy; from a few baby steps, to walking in the corridor, and out into the world. One year later, Ajji again reigned supreme in her home.

Chronic pelvic pain

Ms AD: This chronic pelvic pain patient came in 2005 with excruciating pain between the pubic bone and the ischial tuberosity ("sit bones"). The problem started two years earlier in the US after Bartholin's abscess drainage at the vaginal entrance without anaesthesia, which her student insurance did not cover. The inadequate, unsuccessful, and extremely painful procedure left her in constant discomfort despite two subsequent procedures under anaesthesia. Exploratory surgery in Mumbai revealed that the tentacles of infection had spread across her perineum with the three openings of urethra, vagina, and anus. Post-operative bleeding necessitated blood transfusions and another surgery to staunch the bleeding. These repeated traumata after a year of festering infection culminated in severe neuropathic pain, unresponsive to pain killers and neuromodulators. She could not stand, sit, or even lie down and internal examination was impossible. She had already consulted several doctors with no relief.

Her normal blood counts ruled out infection. It was explained to her that the immediate priority was to stop the pain with CNB of the terminal spinal cord inside the tailbone to quieten the irritated inflamed perineal nerves. She readily agreed for caudal epidural catheter placement (Figure 48).

Her response was a dramatic and gratifying ability to sit, stand, and walk normally. She was thrilled to finally sleep soundly. The following week saw her steadily become pain-free and her bubbly effervescent personality emerged from the anxious, harried persona of the first consultation. After the catheter removal, she had a pinpoint of pain between the vagina and the anus, which responded to Botox. At this juncture the importance of muscles and neuromyopathy was in its infancy; hence the administration of the Botox injection did not have the current Ashirvad understanding or sophistication at that time. Fortunately for AD, the pain ceased completely, and she continued to lead a happy married life. However, it was with the next patient (Ms R), who came because her father was AD's doctor who gave the deeper insights about chronic pelvic pain.

Painful bladder syndrome

Ms R studying law in UK, had severe interstitial cystitis ICS/painful bladder syndrome (PBS) for five years since she was 17, after suspected (but not proven) urinary bladder tuberculosis. She was unresponsive to repeated bladder dilatation, dimethyl sulfoxide (DMSO) instillation, amitriptyline (neuromodulator) and Pentosan polysulphate sodium (Elmiron), to restore the mucus layer that protects the bladder wall from urinary bacteria and irritant chemicals.

Her shrunken bladder could hold only 50 ml (normal female bladder capacity is 400–600 ml) of urine. The continuous lower abdominal and perineal pain, frequent painful urination, worsened at night. After straining one hour to pass 30–40 ml of burning urine that refused to come out, she would drop into exhausted sleep, only to repeat the process an hour later. Intermittent severe perineal shocks radiated to her ankles, particularly on sexual arousal.

- Living alone in England, this terrible body-mind trauma made her despondent, but she was strong willed, hanging in there, determined to go on.
- She spoke in an emotionless monotone, refusing eye contact, hostile and contemptuous towards all doctors.
- The whole family's morale was affected; the mother had the 'luxury' of continuous silent crying, but the equally loving and distressed father had no such outlet.

Available literature revealed that there was very limited knowledge or awareness of this unusual condition. Even bladder removal surgery would not relieve the pain, which would recur in the new bladder made out of the intestines. There were too many grey areas, with no solution in sight. Neither neuropathy nor interventions were mentioned in literature. The nerves controlling urination, sympathetic and parasympathetic functions were mentioned but surprisingly, not the nerves subserving bladder pain. The logical approach was to target the entire bladder nerve supply with a continuous caudal block and a lumbar SGB to reduce possible SMP. Cessation of pain would hopefully unwind five years of severe pain input and CNS sensitization right up to her brain.

The family gave informed consent despite uncertainties regarding the success in reducing the difficulties in urinary frequency and voiding, the risk of epidural catheter infection, with a potentially life-threatening complication like meningitis, and the need for administering continuous antibiotics while the catheter was *in situ*.

The patient, R, had extreme skin hypersensitivity to cleansing her back (hyperesthesia, allodynia) numbing injection and needle advancement (hyperalgesia). Disheartened, she wanted to cancel the caudal CNB, particularly after an ineffective lumbar sympathetic block. Fortunately, her father, who was attending the procedure convinced her not to give up. A fluoroscopy-guided catheter tip was placed between the S2 and S4 nerves (Figure 48). The catheter was tunnelled 10 cm away from its skin entry site to safeguard against infection and accidental expulsion. Continuous 2 m/hour infusion of 0.0625 per cent anaesthetic bupivacaine reduced R's abdominal and perineal pain by 80 per cent overnight, without interfering with the urination/bladder continence. She was so elated to sleep through the night after five years that she convinced her pathologist father, for continuing CNB with weekly blood count monitoring. By three weeks, the urinary frequency decreased significantly, voiding 300 ml once in 2–3 hours, showing that the shrunken bladder of ICS was not an irreversible organic feature and could expand. Being pain-free became her new norm with personality changes like smiling, laughing, and vivacious talking.

Her feedback was vital and valuable at this stage and proved to be very objective. Persistent voiding difficulties, straining and pain indicated some obstruction, but where? Previous cystoscopies by senior urologists reported no obstructions. Constant puzzling about this problem, opened a Pandora's box of questions:

- Normally when the detrusor (the bladder wall muscle) contracts to expel urine, the urethral sphincter cooperates by relaxing for smooth urination. Was her sphincter refusing to cooperate, by paradoxically contracting instead of relaxing, to close the urethral opening to cause obstruction?

- Had the suspected bladder tuberculosis reversed this detrusor/sphincter coordination?

- Would other bladder infections also cause similar problems?
- Was the pelvic floor, a musculofascial hammock extending from the coccyx (tailbone) at the back to the pubic arch in front, contracted, causing this intermittent obstruction with constant discomfort?

Paradoxical dynamic urethral obstruction, which logically explained the burning and the discomfort during and after micturition would be missed during cystoscopy but could be documented during urodynamic flowmetry. But R flatly refused saying, "Doctor, I hate urodynamic study! you can treat me for anything you suspect, but no tortures like urodynamic study."

The very hesitant suggestion of a trial of DN to relax the urethral sphincter was eagerly accepted. R was positively enthusiastic about any treatment to reduce her straining. She asserted, "Doctor, go right ahead." With pain relief from the caudal catheter, which she was holding onto like a lifeline, very cautious DN around the urethra was successfully conducted. The next day, a jubilant R exclaimed, "I don't know what you did nor what the science behind it was, but I am much better!" Although the obstruction decreased with DN, worries about its recurrence after she returned to the UK, remained.

Urologists inject botulinum toxin (botox) through a cystoscope to relax the bladder wall but that would not relax the sphincter, which was obviously the problem. There was no mention in pain literature at the time (in 2006) of Botox injection into the sphincter and the pelvic floor muscles in ICS/PBS. Since DN helped her, this was the logical treatment for R, although there was a risk of urine leakage with an excess of Botox. With great confidence, R said, "Doctor, I trust your hunches and judgements absolutely and have no fear when I am with you. If I leak, I will simply wear a diaper! After all, Botox wears off in four-to-five months." The family was absolutely cooperative, and the father confirmed, "Doctor, it is not as if the scientifically accepted treatments have helped her! It is only after your unorthodox treatment that we see our daughter smile in the morning after a good night's sleep. So, please go ahead."

Anxiety was paramount at this juncture of treading a completely unknown territory. The plan was to use only 100 units of Botox. But the extreme resistance by the rock-hard muscles to needle penetration necessitated a higher Botox dose to reduce her struggle to pass urine. Fortunately, 300 units proved to be the right decision, completely reducing her obstruction and the clitoral pain without any adverse effects. Finally, R was happy! But the fear and hesitation about vaginal examination remained. After two failed attempts when she apologized, she had to be reminded that she had no real problem, but she had to stop being a brat in her own interest despite her deep-seated fear and psychological issues regarding internal examination. Looking shocked she promised, "Tomorrow I will not be a brat." True to her word, she permitted the examination realizing in the process, that indeed it was more her fear than actual pain and that nothing prevented her from having a normal life. She returned to the UK, symptom-and phobia-free.

She required repeat Botox injections at steadily increasing intervals of 6–12–18 months and none after the last injection in 2013. She is happily married and works as a solicitor in London. She is still cautious about what she eats since some foods worsen her symptoms.

This sharp young lady, despite her extreme problems, anxiety, and frustration, that had so radically altered her personality, did not waste time feeling sorry for herself, bemoaning her fate. She just focused on getting through life, one day at a time. By constantly pushing for better results, she is responsible for the genesis of out-of-the-box concepts on ICS, which have benefited 25 other women and 15 men since then.

The collective understanding from all these patients:

- Infection or trauma can cause/worsen pelvic floor muscle spasm, particularly urethral, anal sphincters and vagina with genitourinary or rectal obstructive symptoms and coccigodynia.

- Some people seem to tighten their perineum when stressed, be it personal, professional performance anxiety, or whatever, leading eventually to pelvic floor muscle spasm.

- The obstruction and painful straining cause excessive bladder pressure leading to trabeculations and Hunner's ulcers. These cystoscopy findings are diagnostic of ICS/PBS.

- Constant struggle, discomfort and burning pain cause peripheral and central sensitization.

- ICS has two distinct components. A primary obstructive problem that leads to a neuropathic pain problem both of which have to be addressed simultaneously for ICS reversal (Chapter 2, Reference 8).

- Mild cases require only neuromodulators and/or USGDN. Others may require Caudal epidural CNB + Botox + USGDN.

• Other pelvic/urogenital pains in both men and women and coccygodynia also respond to similar treatment.

This innovative therapy along with patient education about the aggravators, cognitive behavioural therapy (CBT), yoga, and *pranayama* to reduce "traffic on the expressway" between the mind and the pelvic floor has stood the test of time. After recovery from neuropathic and obstructive symptoms, patients return only because of exacerbations caused by urinary infections, stress/anxiety. USGDN significantly reduces the Botox requirement over the years.

Finally, all patients of ICS/PBS and chronic pelvic pains owe a huge debt of gratitude to Ms R and her family, without whose absolute trust and cooperation it would not have been possible to develop this treatment.

Where there's a will, there's a way

A 26-year-old student, AP, suffered with back pain since 2003. A skateboard injury in 2004 triggered severe radiating calf pain, which settled with bed rest, physiotherapy, and chiropraxy. A year later, a tennis game triggered L5-S1 disc prolapse. Despite oral steroids, traction, one blind, two X-ray-guided epidural steroid injections, and microdiscectomy in April 2006, and opioids (which he fortunately stopped), did not relieve his pain. He took a fourth epidural to travel to India. He was at Ashirvad in December 2006 with pain which limited him to standing for 5 minutes, walking 15 minutes, sitting 1 hour, lying supine 1–2 minutes. His back had only 10^0 flexion/extension and extremely tight hamstrings and adductors. He consented to Racz adhesiolysis for dissolving the scar around the L5 nerve root, and USGDN.

The recovery: Radio-opaque dye showed a surgical scar obstructing the right S1 foramen. Hyaluronidase injections, which selectively dissolve fibrous tissue, through Racz catheter over the next two days; a 40-mg steroid injection reduced his leg pain by 50 per cent. Thereafter, USGDN and Botox released all the taut and tight muscles around his ramrod stiff spine, adductors, hamstrings, and leg muscles. He was now walking for one hour, using public transport, and sitting for two-to-three hours without pain. Movements which were like a 70-year-old's reverted to those of the 26-year-old that he was.

He later wrote from the US that daily physiotherapy for three hours was integral to his life to maintain the restored muscle equilibrium. The following year he had gone off all medications with pain-free, full range, back movements and the erstwhile crippling pains were forgotten.

Care for the back

The human back is unique in its functionality. Nature originally designed the spine for quadrupeds with stability divided between four legs. An erect posture, in human beings with a high centre of gravity balanced on the narrow base of the legs, requires stabilization by the adductor muscles and hamstrings to support the torso. This puts tremendous strain on the lower back while standing, walking, and running. Most of the spinal cord is protected by a bony back canal which is almost continuous in the front with the individual vertebrae separated by intervertebral discs while at the back it forms a bony arch with a strong set of ligaments between the bones. This arrangement provides enough access for the nerves to leave and enter the spinal cord at various levels and allows a tremendous but variable amount of mobility to different parts of the spine.

The intervertebral disc is fluid in the centre (nucleus pulposus), which is enclosed by a tough annulus fibrosus to form an oval which is like a jelly ball which buffers all the spine movements admirably. This disc has no blood supply. It gets its nutrition by repetitive bending forward and backward movements.

Daily yoga type flexion/extension stretches like front-to-back (*Surya Namaskar* Figure 45), side-to-side (*Chandra Namaskar*), and twists keep the back muscles toned and supple. Exercise prevents premature spine degeneration that weakens the annulus fibrosus of the disc, which can tear and cause prolapsed disc. The intervertebral discs, which depend on repetitive flexion/extension to draw nourishment from the surrounding fluid, got none in this man's daily routine (Figure 49).

Sitting cross-legged stretches the adductors (inner thigh muscles), Psoas (attaches vertebral front to the upper thigh) and stabilizes the back to optimally balance the body weight on the ischial tuberosities in the buttocks (Figure 49). He would study long hours sitting slouched or wedged into a fixed position in a chair without getting up. Stretching every hour and walking, which works the left and right sides of the back optimally, is important. Prolonged sitting gradually shortens the back muscles, adductors, hamstrings, and calf muscles. Spasm of the powerful back muscles (Figure 28, Chapter 3, Figure 49) squeezes the vertebrae together to pressurize the discs (causing tears, prolapse) and facets (causing arthritis). Shortened adductor muscles generate stress

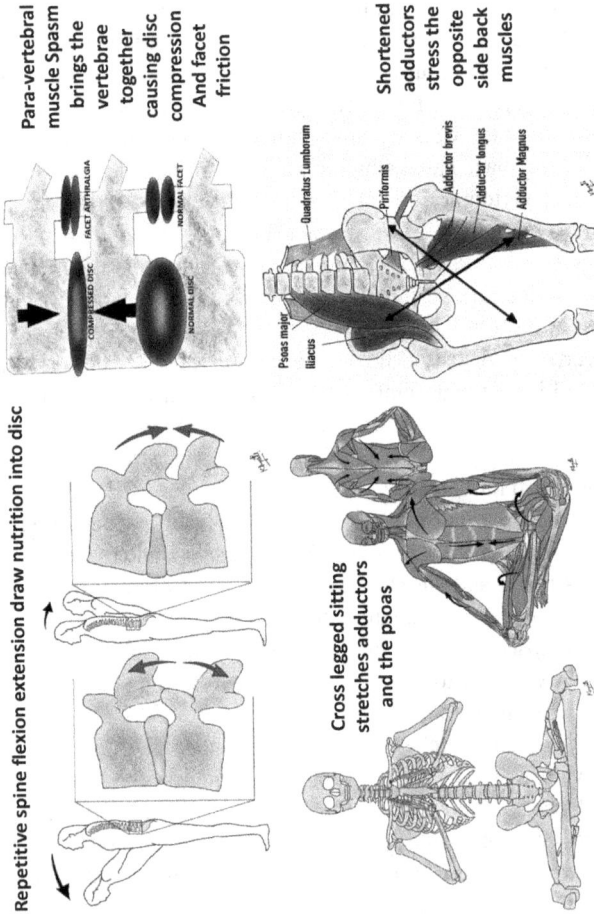

Figure 49. Sitting cross legged is a very stable position and also stretches the adductors and the psoas muscle to keep the back supple and healthy.

and pain in Quadratus lumborum, erector spinae, and Psoas muscles of the opposite side (Figure 49). Shortened hamstrings cause back arching.

His deconditioned back muscles were further subjected to various shears and pressures of vigorous sports, skate boarding, gym, tennis *without* the mandatory prior stretching or later cooldown. Gym-type exercises, where the back is fixed for lifting heavy weights, stress the disc by raising the intradiscal pressure and running causes degenerative changes in spine, hip, knees and ankles over the years. Therefore, the skateboard fall precipitated his undernourished desiccated disc to herniate!

Treatment was suboptimal because, to address the intervertebral disc, the steroid should reach the front but a blind epidural deposits it at the back compartment of the epidural space without dye-spread confirmation. Advise on back health, exercises, or physiotherapy was not provided.

Neither the epidurals nor the surgery addressed the painful muscles, instrumental in causing the disc to prolapse since they maintain the overall back health and mechanics. Since muscles are the most important contributors to pain it is but natural that patients continue to be in pain. Additionally, the multifidus muscle (essential for normal back mechanics) is removed in back surgery to allow access to the disc. USGDN relieves all these accumulated pains from before the surgery and those secondary to post-surgical neuromyopathy. USGDN also released micro doses of platelet-rich plasma into the scar to regenerate the muscles. Finally, USGDN, Botox, and diligent physiotherapy restored the elasticity to the back and limb muscles by addressing the multitudes of MTrPs remaining after failed back surgery.

A pain specialist's pain

All was right in VS's career of busy anaesthesiology till 2005. But a swollen middle finger brought her world crashing down as a harbinger of rheumatoid arthritis (RA) at age 33.

Hydroxychloroquine, regular daily analgesics, oral and subcutaneous methotrexate at six months, and steroids thereafter gave no relief. The following year was filled with pain and side-effects of methotrexate and hydroxychloroquine—severe anaemia, retinal pigmentation, and visual problems. The worst was the steroid, which predisposed her to tuberculosis with pleural effusion. Life was turned upside down for this doctor who had become the patient; all her dreams of further education, successful career, and having a family disappeared because of this disease with lifelong pain and disability, which she felt she was destined to suffer alone.

Unable to take medication, she vainly tried ayurveda, homeopathy, physiotherapy, acupressure, acupuncture, and massage for the fast-advancing painful RA. Replacement of both hips and knees in 2011–2012 relieved the pain and helped her through what she calls "one horrible phase of life". She could work comfortably again but only for two years! the pains recurred in the joints of shoulders, elbows, hands, ankles and toes, with a constantly high inflammatory marker, CRP levels of 40 (N = < 5). While life and work continued, the big question was what to do next.

In 2018, Ms VS joined a six-day USGDN workshop at Ashirvad, to learn/relearn cadaver lab anatomy with all the new perspectives on pain being taught. She professed to be amazed with all this learning and impressed at hearing the testimonials given to her on interviewing a number of satisfied Ashirvad patients with rare problems like Interstitial cystitis, CRPS, neuropathic, and cancer pains. She was surprised to see that a few patients were from the USA, UK, and Hongkong with post-op knee and hip joint pains. So much so she decided to get the Ashirvad treatment herself.

Her treatment started with PRF of the nerves of the knee and shoulder joints and USGDN of all the muscles in the pain areas. Consistent improvement at one month when her warm joints assumed normal temperature, confirming no inflammation, gave her immense hope and confidence to be comfortable, pain-free. Her baseline heart rate, which was always high (100–110/minute) due to continuous pain, dropped to 70–80/minute. She was thrilled with her lowered CRP level of 14!

Ms VS wanted to learn this treatment, which had given her hope for a normal life. She did a three-month AIPMR fellowship and later one-year Pain Management university fellowship, in 2020. She started a pain clinic at BYL Nair hospital in Mumbai adopting the AIPMR approach. She is doing valuable work at this public hospital catering to lower socioeconomic strata, getting amazing results with varieties of pains with very happy and satisfied patients.

Ms VS says that the AIPMR experience changed her life, and now, at age 49 years, in her own words, "I know I am doing something worthwhile that positively influences other lives just as Ashirvad touched my life, when my patients at the Nair pain clinic come back with smiles."

We shall succeed!

Captain M was in the elite anti-terrorist unit of the Indian army in Kashmir. His "never say die" motto reverberated, when in 2012, at age 24, a terrorist's bullet penetrated his L1 vertebra, and exited through the abdomen necessitating immediate abdominal and spine surgery. The powerful rifle-fired bullet created shock waves above and below the entry into the spine, causing extensive spinal cord damage, and left him paralysed below the waist; with a burning electric current-like unbearable pain, called causalgia, preventing daily activities, and more importantly, interfering with his concentration to read the scripture, *Bhagavad Gita,* his only succour in life.

Extensive skin hypersensitivity made the touch of clothing and even a slight breeze unbearable. These problems had remained unresponsive to stem-cell therapy, pain medications, epidural injections, abdominal nerve blocks and mind distraction therapies.

Dr Dua, the pain specialist for the entire armed forces, who knew of Ashirvad work in neuropathic pain referred Captain M in 2014. Since his trunk muscles lacked the strength to hold his spine erect, he had travelled on a stretcher in the ambulance but had moved into a wheelchair for his consultation. Knowing his background information, it was a pleasant surprise to be greeted cheerily by a bright personable young man, sitting crunched up in his Ottobok wheelchair, instead of a dour-faced person on a stretcher.

He reported increased sweating (hyperhydrosis), warmth over the torso and flinching on being touched. Both paralysed legs showed severe muscle wasting and no sensations but for phantom pain in the right leg. He was an exceptional young man with a strong personality who, in an apologetically self-effacing manner, admitted that his pain was an intrusive nuisance. This was his description of causalgia or CRPS-2, one of the most dreaded of pains in all pain literature! Adept at ignoring bodily pains as part of his special forces training, he successfully downplayed his problems even to himself. But spinal cord injury pains are so severe that he had to seek help. Prima facie, causalgia has no definitive treatment. It was explained to him that while there was no guarantee, USGDN procedure for at least two-to-three months could be tried to relieve the pain and hypersensitivity with maybe some functional restoration

A lumbar sympathetic block was conducted on the same day, but there was no improvement. But three USGDN sessions reduced the shocks although the hypersensitivity and burning remained the same. This was enough to make him determined to return and we were determined to do the best for someone who had given his youth and life for his country. A month later, M was admitted on medical leave, into Mumbai's naval hospital with two trusted aides from his own division.

Thus started a treatment, which provided a great learning about the young human body's resilience and the driving ambition of a strong mind to succeed against all odds. The one problem was that this commando was so trained to evade interrogation that he kept skirting around the pain facts. But details of these facts were essential for ensuring proper treatment. Finally, he gave some pain scores, possibly to halt the inquisition! Months later he admitted that pain denial was so deeply ingrained in his psyche that he just could not dwell on his bodily pain. The power of the mind is formidable indeed.

After PRF for his abdominal nerves, and systematic USGDN of the entire torso musculature led to the disappearance of:

- Shocks radiating from the spine down his back.
- Extremely tender abdominal triggers, which used to make him blackout when pressed.
- "Insect-crawling" in his lower back.
- The constant agonizing truncal burning pain and hypersensitivity.
- Most importantly, he could sit up straight without support even in a moving vehicle. With this significant improvement, he could hone his sharpshooting skills for competitive shooting.

A steroid trigger injection+ targeted USGDN on his left chest wall, eliminated the excruciating pain waves therefrom. By this time, he was comfortable enough to discuss his future plans and aspirations. The logical advice was to start working in his old unit to occupy his mind rather than focus on shooting, a boring mechanical activity. He laughed and said, "What? A paralysed guy in special forces! no way!" He dismissed the suggestion that he could possibly shift the work profile to one who plans strategies, or someone who procures special equipment making sure that his buddies get the best. It seemed that with his disability, he obviously loathed returning to a unit where he had been one of the daredevils.

Interestingly, during abdominal USGDN, he reported that something "opened up" in his otherwise numb legs. This defied medical understanding, but trusting his report focused needling of that area was conducted. This approach of modifying the treatment, with the assumption that patients know their bodies better than the treating physician does, had yielded rich dividends in understanding many pain conditions at Ashirvad and it did so now as well. This "opening" sensation was associated with sonography demonstration of some mild twitches in his thigh muscles. In his typical M fashion, He said, "Ma'am, give me even the smallest twitches in my legs and I shall make life hell for them till they move."

USGDN procedure of his wasted lower limbs was done with a vague notion that maybe, the muscles might regain some life. Sure enough, the muscles in his legs became firmer with the treatment, gained some bulk increasing the limb girth by 1–2 inches and assumed normal contours. The microtrauma from needling was probably releasing blood platelets into the muscles to act as a local regenerative treatment. This regeneration was an unexpected bonus, which helped him to stand up with callipers and attempt moving with a walker (Figure 50). The first time when he stood up to his six-feet height, he looked so handsome and well-built that it was a pity that he could not do it all the time! But then one can't argue with fate. This was what his parents, a simple young couple, who came to meet the doctor who was making their son stand and walk, had to sorrowfully accept.

Three months later, M was walking 45–60 minutes with a walker and callipers; he was able to travel through Mumbai traffic in an ordinary taxi; and most importantly, his original buoyant and exuberant personality resurfaced. Many girls flocked around him wishing to become his girlfriend. But M was no fool, he enjoyed their company, keeping them at arm's length!

He returned to active duty and shooting practice. At the six-month check-up, he shared something interesting. Usually marksmen stand and shoot, but he would sit, twist his torso sideways, hold up a 1-kg pistol at a 90° angle at the shoulder and then shoot. This would be an extremely uncomfortable position to hold for anyone, and for someone with paralysed legs and causalgia around the trunk, it required tremendous endurance and one-pointed focus! To maintain such a position his torso muscles would be screaming. But M being M, he declared breezily that he practiced four hours non-stop! Hats off to such determination and courage! He just asked for USGDN to eliminate his head and neck pains, brain fog, and the concentration issues and returned to his practice. His

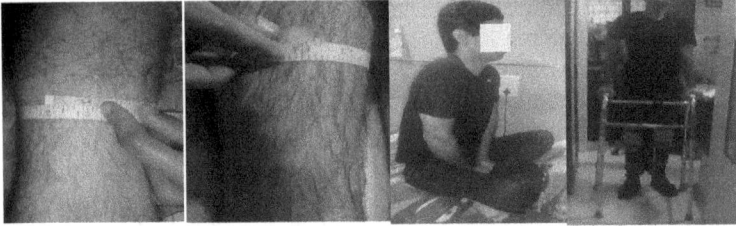

Figure 50. Left: 11/2" increase in thigh girth, normal hair and contour. Middle: Sitting without support. Right: Walking with callipers and walker.

morale was high he was happy and on February 29, 2015, he celebrated his 28th birthday at Ashirvad.

M set several national pistol shooting records. He also cleared his departmental exam with flying colours to become a Major in 2016. Most happily for him, he returned to his old unit as a procurement officer in 2019. He brought his charming wife to meet us in December 2021. He continues to walk an hour daily, exercises regularly and leads a very active life. He visits the clinic during his annual leave for a reunion and also gets USGDN done for any bothersome issues.

Index

For Product Safety Concerns and Information please contact our EU
representative GPSR@taylorandfrancis.com
Taylor & Francis Verlag GmbH, Kaufingerstraße 24, 80331 München, Germany